The Little Black Book of

Pediatrics

Series Editor: Daniel K. Onion

Chiedza G. Jokonya, MD, MRCPCH
Maine Dartmouth Family Medicine
Residency Program
Augusta, Maine

Sydney R. Sewall, MD, MPH
Kennebec Pediatrics
Augusta, Maine

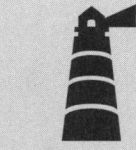

JONES & BARTLETT
LEARNING

World Headquarters

Jones & Bartlett Learning
40 Tall Pine Drive
Sudbury, MA 01776
978-443-5000
info@jblearning.com
www.jblearning.com

Jones & Bartlett Learning Canada
6339 Ormindale Way
Mississauga, Ontario L5V 1J2
Canada

Jones & Bartlett Learning
International
Barb House, Barb Mews
London W6 7PA
United Kingdom

Jones & Bartlett Learning books and products are available through most bookstores and online booksellers. To contact Jones & Bartlett Learning directly, call 800-832-0034, fax 978-443-8000, or visit our website, www.jblearning.com.

Substantial discounts on bulk quantities of Jones & Bartlett Learning publications are available to corporations, professional associations, and other qualified organizations. For details and specific discount information, contact the special sales department at Jones & Bartlett Learning via the above contact information or send an email to specialsales@jblearning.com.

The authors, editor, and publisher have made every effort to provide accurate information. However, they are not responsible for errors, omissions, or for any outcomes related to the use of the contents of this book and take no responsibility for the use of the products and procedures described. Treatments and side effects described in this book may not be applicable to all people; likewise, some people may require a dose or experience a side effect that is not described herein. Drugs and medical devices are discussed that may have limited availability controlled by the Food and Drug Administration (FDA) for use only in a research study or clinical trial. Research, clinical practice, and government regulations often change the accepted standard in this field. When consideration is being given to use of any drug in the clinical setting, the healthcare provider or reader is responsible for determining FDA status of the drug, reading the package insert, and reviewing prescribing information for the most up-to-date recommendations on dose, precautions, and contraindications, and determining the appropriate usage for the product. This is especially important in the case of drugs that are new or seldom used.

Production Credits
Senior Acquisitions Editor: Nancy Anastasi Duffy
Editorial Assistant: Sara Cameron
Associate Production Editor: Laura Almozara
Marketing Manager: Rebecca Rockel
V.P., Manufacturing and Inventory Control:
  Therese Connell

Project Management: Thistle Hill Publishing
  Services, LLC
Composition: Dedicated Business Solutions
Cover Design: Anne Spencer/Kristin E. Parker
Cover Image: © Photos.com
Printing and Binding: Malloy, Inc.
Cover Printing: Malloy, Inc.

Library of Congress Cataloging-in-Publication Data
Jokonya, Chiedza G.
    The little black book of pediatrics / Chiedza G. Jokonya, Sydney R. Sewall.
        p.; cm. — (Little black book series)
Includes bibliographical references and index.
    ISBN-13: 978-0-7637-5446-4 (pbk.)
    ISBN-10: 0-7637-5446-3 (pbk.)
    1. Pediatrics—Handbooks, manuals, etc. I. Sewall, Sydney R. II.
Title. III. Series: Little black book series.
    [DNLM: 1. Pediatrics—Handbooks. WS 39]
    RJ48.J595 2012
    618.92—dc22

                                                                    2010050877

6048

Printed in the United States of America
15 14 13 12 11   10 9 8 7 6 5 4 3 2 1

Dedication

This book is dedicated to my father, Tichaona Joseph Jokonya (1933–2006), and my mother, Winifrieda Jokonya. Their love, guidance, and nurturing made me the person I am today.

—CGJ

To Joan Marson, RN, Case Manager at MaineGeneral Health, whose dedication to her many animals is only exceeded by her caring efforts toward helping our most needy patients.

—SRS

Contents

Preface

Syd Sewell and I were asked by Dan Onion to contribute to a pediatric edition of the Little Black Book (LBB) series. Our book generally follows the format of the LBB series, with the goal of providing an overview of common topics in pediatrics with embedded references that support the text and discussing controversies or current research into new management modalities. Our target audiences are physicians in general, as well as pediatricians and primary care clinicians in training.

I'd like to express my thanks to Dan Onion, who acted as a mentor through the process of writing this book and for his valuable advice in reviewing the book for me. I'd also like to thank Karen Gershman and Misha Lazerow, who also helped review chapters of the book.

Chiedza G. Jokonya

Medical Abbreviations

×	times	ARM	anorectal manometry
μg	microgram	ART	antiretroviral therapy
		ASA	aminosalicylic acid
AAP	American Academy of Pediatrics	AST	aspartate transferase
		ATN	acute tubular necrosis
ABCs	airway, breathing, circulation in resuscitation	AVN	atrioventricular node
		BCG	Bacille Calmette-Guérin
ABPA	allergic bronchopulmonary aspergillosis	BGL	blood glucose level
ACEI	angiotensin-converting enzyme inhibitor	BMI	body mass index
		BMT	bone marrow transplant
ADH	antidiuretic hormone	BP	blood pressure
ADHD	attention deficit hyperactivity disorder	BT	bleeding time
AFB	acid-fast bacilli	BUN	blood urea nitrogen
AIDS	acquired immune deficiency syndrome	CAH	congenital adrenal hyperplasia
ALL	acute lymphoblastic leukemia	cAMP	cyclic adenosine monophosphate
ALT	alanine transferase	CBC	complete blood count
AML	acute myeloblastic leukemia	CBC/D	complete blood count/differential
AMS	altered mental status	CD	Crohn's disease
ANA	antinuclear antibody	CDC	Centers for Disease Control and Prevention
AOM	acute otitis media		
AP	anteroposterior Xray		
ARAS	ascending reticular activating system	CF	cystic fibrosis

CFTR	cystic fibrosis trans-membrane conductance regulator (gene)	ERCP	endoscopic retrograde cholangiopancre-atography
CHF	congestive heart failure	ESR	erythrocyte sedimenta-tion rate
Cl	chloride	ESRD	end-stage renal disease
CMV	cytomegalovirus	ETEC	enterotoxigenic *Escherichia coli*
CNS	central nervous system		
CPK	creatinine phosphokinase	FDA	Food and Drug Administration
CRP	C-reactive protein	FHT	fetal heart tones/tracing
CSF	cerebrospinal fluid		
CT	computerized tomography	FSGS	focal segmental glomerulosclerosis
CXR	chest Xray	FSH	follicle-stimulating hormone
d	day(s)	FTT	failure to thrive
DIC	disseminated intravas-cular coagulation		
DIP	distal interphalangeal	GBM	glomerular basement membrane
DKA	diabetes ketoacidosis	GBS	Guillain-Barré syndrome
DM	diabetes mellitus		
DMD	Duchenne muscular dystrophy	GC	*Neisseria gonorrhoeae*
DUB	dysfunctional uterine bleeding	GERD	gastroesophageal reflux disease
dx	diagnosis	GFR	glomerular filtration rate
EBV	Epstein-Barr virus	GH	growth hormone
EEG	electroencephalogram	gi	gastrointestinal
EKG	electrocardiogram	GN	glomerulonephritis
ELISA	enzyme-linked immu-nosorbent assay	GU	genitourinary
EMG	electromyelogram	H + P	history and physical
ENT	ear nose and throat	HAART	highly active antiretro-viral therapy

hb/hgb	hemoglobin	kg	kilogram
HbA_{1c}	glycosylated hemoglobin (major fraction)	KOH	potassium hydroxide
HCO_3	bicarbonate	L	liter
HIV	human immunodeficiency virus	LBW	low birthweight
		LDH	lactate dehydrogenase
HPV	human papillomavirus	LDL	low-density lipoprotein
HR	heart rate	LFT	liver function test
hr	hour(s)	LH	luteinizing hormone
hx	history	LLQ	left lower quadrant
		LP	lumbar puncture
I&D	incision and drainage	LV	left ventricle
I&O	intake and output		
IBD	inflammatory bowel disease	M:F	male-to-female ratio
		MCGN	minimal change glomerulonephritis
ICU	intensive care unit		
IDA	iron deficiency anemia	MCUG	micturating cystourethrogram
IDDM	infant of diabetic mother		
		MCV	mean cell volume
Ig	immunoglobulin	mg	milligram
IL	interleukin	$MgSO_4$	magnesium sulphate
im	intramuscular	mL	milliliter
IRT	immunoreactive trypsinogen	MMR	measles, mumps, rubella
IU	international unit	MR	mental retardation
IUGR	intrauterine growth restriction	MRI	magnetic resonance imaging
IV	intravenous	MRSA	methicillin-resistant *Staphylococcus aureus*
IVDU	IV drug user		
IVIG	IV immunoglobulin	MTCT	mother-to-child transmission
IVP	intravenous pyelogram		
		Na	sodium
JIA	juvenile idiopathic arthritis	NBICU	newborn intensive care unit
		NG	nasogastric
K+	potassium		

NGT	nasogastric tube	PUD	peptic ulcer disease
NPO	nothing by mouth	PWS	port wine stain
NS	normal saline		
NSAID	nonsteroidal anti-inflammatory drug	q	every
		r/o	rule out
OME	otitis media with effusion	rbc	red blood cell
		RLQ	right lower quadrant
ORS	oral rehydration solution	RLS	restless leg syndrome
		RMSF	Rocky Mountain spotted fever
ORT	oral rehydration therapy	RNC	radionucleotide cystogram
OTC	over the counter	RSB	rectal suction biopsy
PBS	peripheral blood smear	RSV	respiratory syncytial virus
PCOS	polycystic ovary syndrome	RTA	renal tubular acidosis
PCP	*Pneumocystis carinii*	RUQ	right upper quadrant
PCR	polymerase chain reaction	RV	right ventricle
		rx	treatment
PICU	pediatric intensive care unit	S+S	signs and symptoms
PID	pelvic inflammatory disease	sc	subcutaneous
		SCD	sickle cell disease
po	per os; orally	SHBG	sex hormone-binding globulin
PPD	purified protein derivative	si	signs
PPI	protein pump inhibitor	SLE	systemic lupus erythematosus
PSGN	poststreptococcal glomerulonephritis	SLIT	sublingual immunotherapy
pt	patient	SMA	spinal muscular atrophy
PT	ProTime		
PTH	parathyroid hormone	SOB	short of breath
PTSD	posttraumatic stress disorder	SSRI	selective serotonin reuptake inhibitor
PTT	partial thromboplastin time		

SSSS	staphylococcus scalded skin syndrome	UA	urinalysis
STI	sexually transmitted infection	UC	ulcerative colitis
		UGI	upper gastrointestinal
sx	symptoms	URI	upper respiratory (tract) infection
TB	tuberculosis	UTI	urinary tract infection
TDD	total daily dose	VCUG	voiding cystourethrogram
TGV	transposition of the great vessels	VDRL	Venereal Disease Research Laboratory
TLC	therapeutic lifestyle change		
TMJ	temporomandibular joint	WCC	white blood cell count
		WHO	World Health Organization
TPN	total parenteral nutrition	wk	week
TSH	thyroid-stimulating hormone	WPW	Wolff-Parkinson-White syndrome
TSI	thyroid-stimulating immunoglobulin	wt	weight
TSS	toxic shock syndrome	yr	year(s)

Journal Abbreviations

Acad Emerg Med	Academic Emergency Medicine
Am Fam Phys	American Family Physician
Am J Clin Nutr	American Journal of Clinical Nutrition
Am J Hum Genet	American Journal of Human Genetics
Am J Med Genet	American Journal of Medical Genetics
Am J Obstet Gynecol	American Journal of Obstetrics and Gynecology
Am J Respir Crit Care Med	American Journal of Respiratory and Critical Care Medicine
Am J Surg	American Journal of Surgery
Ann Emerg Med	Annals of Emergency Medicine
Ann Intern Med	Annals of Internal Medicine
Ann NY Acad Sci	Annals of the New York Academy of Sciences
Arch Dermatol	Archives of Dermatology
Arch Dis Child	Archives of Diseases of Childhood
Arch Pediatr Adolesc Med	Archives of Pediatric Adolescent Medicine
Brain Dev	Brain Development
Cancer	Cancer
Circulation	Circulation
Clin Infect Dis	Clinical Infectious Diseases
Clin J Sport Med	Clinical Journal of Sports Medicine
Clin Pediatr	Clinical Pediatrics
Cochrane Database Syst Rev	Cochrane Database of Systemic Reviews
Crit Care Med	Critical Care Medicine

Dermatol Clin	Dermatology Clinic
Diabet Med	Diabetes Medicine
Diabetes Care	Diabetes Care
Emerg Med J	Emergency Medicine Journal
Eur J Pediatr	European Journal of Pediatrics
J Am Acad Dermatol	Journal of the American Academy of Dermatology
J Am Soc Nephrol	Journal of the American Society of Nephrology
J Clin Endocrinol Metab	Journal of Clinical Endocrinology and Metabolism
J Clin Oncol	Journal of Clinical Oncology
J Infect Dis	Journal of Infectious Diseases
J Pediatr	Journal of Pediatrics
J Pediatr Endocrinol Metab	Journal of Pediatric Endocrinology and Metabolism
J Pediatr Gastroenterol Nutr	Journal of Pediatric Gastroenterology and Nutrition
J Pediatr Hematol Oncol	Journal of Pediatric Hematology and Oncology
J Rheumatol	Journal of Rheumatology
J Urol	Journal of Urology
J Vasc Surg	Journal of Vascular Surgery
JAMA	Journal of the American Medical Association
Lancet	Lancet
Med Pediatr Oncol	Medical and Pediatric Oncology
N Engl J Med	New England Journal of Medicine
Pediatr Dermatol	Pediatric Dermatology
Pediatr Infect Dis J	The Pediatric Infectious Disease Journal

Pediatr J Neurol	Pediatric Journal of Neurology
Pediatr Rev	Pediatrics in Review
Pediatrics	Pediatrics
Postgrad Med J	Postgraduate Medicine Journal
Sleep Med	Sleep Medicine
Soc Sci Med	Social Science & Medicine

Notice

We have made every attempt to summarize accurately and concisely a multitude of references. However, we must remind our readers that times and medical knowledge change, transcription errors are always possible, and crucial details are necessarily omitted whenever such a comprehensive distillation is attempted in a limited space. And the primary purpose of this compilation is to cite literature on various sides of controversial issues, knowing that where "truth" lies is usually difficult to discern. Thus, we cannot guarantee that every bit of information is absolutely accurate or complete. Readers should affirm that cited recommendations are still reasonable by reading the original articles and checking other sources, including local consultants as well as recent literature, before applying them.

Drugs and medical devices are discussed that may have limited availability, controlled by the Food and Drug Administration (FDA) for use only in research study or clinical trials. The drug information presented has been derived from reference sources, recently published data, and pharmaceutical tests. Research, clinical practice, and government regulations often change the accepted standard in this field. When consideration is given to the use of any drug in the clinical setting, the clinician or reader is responsible for determining the FDA status of the drug; reading the package insert and prescribing information for the most up-to-date recommendations on dose, precautions, and contraindications; and determining the appropriate use for the product. This is especially important in the case of drugs that are new or seldom used.

Chapter 1

Emergency Pediatrics

1.1   Acute Life-Threatening Event

General Ref

- *Pediatr Rev* 2007;28

Cause

- Multifactorial
- Previously "apnea" or "near-miss sudden infant death syndrome (SIDS)"

Epidem

- Separate entity from true SIDS (*Pediatrics* 2003;111:914).
- Estimated 2.46 per 1000 white births (*AAP Grand Rounds* 2005;13:55).
- Many cases represent benign events with overreaction by caretaker.
- Over half remain idiopathic after complete workup (*Pediatr Rev* 2002;23).

S+S

- Infant "not breathing" or "choking" with breathing, color change, decreased muscle tone.
- Sx can be first sign of respiratory syncytial virus (RSV) or systemic bacterial infection, but more commonly infant appears well on presentation; can be symptom of Munchausen by proxy or abuse.

Lab

- Directed by H+P, such as RSV or pertussis testing
  - In "occult" cases, no single test adds much information.
  - If admitted for observation and monitoring, get CBC/D, electrolytes, UA, culture.
  - Septic appearance warrants blood culture and lumbar puncture (LP).
  - Unrecognized inborn errors of metabolism are extremely rare, but consider if infant acidotic without explanation or unusual family hx.
  - EKG for QT.
  - Covert video screening applied in extreme circumstances.

Xray

- Chest Xray; consider barium swallow (and/or pH probe if available).
- Consider child abuse; some recommend CNS imaging for all (*AAP Grand Rounds* 2004;11:3) unless alternative dx obvious.

Rx

- Home monitoring *not* recommended (*AAP*, 2003)
  - Rx triggering condition.
  - Association with gastroesophageal reflux (GER) is controversial, but use H_2 blockers if suspected.
  - Discontinue smoking; reinforce "back to sleep."
  - Having parents know basic life support may give them confidence.

Commentary

- First determine if infant is "sick" or "well," and treat sick infants emergently.
  - If infant appears fine, usual course is admission for observation.
  - Set parameters on any monitor to avoid frequent false alarms.
  - Period of observation is the most helpful "test."

1.2   Altered Mental Status

General Ref

- *Am J Emerg Med* 2002;20:613–617
- *Clin Pediatr Emerg Med* 2003;4:171–178
- *Pediatr Rev* 2006;27:331–337

Cause

The mnemonic AEIOU TIPS is useful to categorize major cause of altered mental status (AMS) in children:

A: alcohol, abuse of substances
E: electrolyte abnormalities, endocrine, epilepsy, encephalopathy
I: intussusception, insulin
O: overdose, oxygen deficiency
U: uremia
T: trauma, tumor, temperature irregularities
I: infection
P: poisons, psychiatric conditions
S: shock, stroke, space-occupying lesions

Epidem

- Different cause more common at different ages.
- Infection most common cause of AMS.
- DKA most common metabolic disorder causing AMS.
- Rate of traumatic injury increases with age.

Pathophys

- Normal regulation of the cycle of wakefulness to sleep is controlled by the ARAS, a brainstem structure sometimes called the "sleep center."
- AMS occurs from either localized abnormalities of the ARAS, global CNS dysfunction, or diffuse dysfunction of the cerebral hemispheres.

S+S

- A good H+P should help elucidate possible cause.
- Symptoms may be gradual (metabolic) or sudden (CNS hemorrhage).
- Fever suggests infection; there may be headache, dizziness, lethargy.

Lab

- Bedside glucose on presentation
- Electrolytes, ABGs
- WBC and differential, blood cultures, LP
- Serum ammonia, LFTs
- Stool guaiac (positive may suggest intussusception)
- EKG

Imaging

- CT scan of head once stable
- EEG and MRI if H+P warrant

Rx

- ABCs of resuscitation.
- 100% oxygen by nonrebreather until adequate oxygenation assured.
- IV access and fluid resuscitation with normal saline.
- Bedside glucose; correct any hypoglycemia.
- Antidotes if H+P suggestive of ingestion (e.g., pinpoint pupils and respiratory depression); in opiate intoxication give naloxone IV.
- Once stable, emergent CT scan head to differentiate structural versus medical problem.

Medical Etiology

- Activated charcoal if toxin ingestion (suspect if no clear etiology in an afebrile toddler or adolescent).

- Further workup to rule out and correct electrolyte or acid-base abnormalities.
- LP (contraindicated if focal signs or clinically unstable), blood cultures, and empirical antibiotics if infection suspected.
- Empirical acyclovir if herpes encephalitis suspected.
- Metabolic panel may suggest inborn errors of metabolism.

Structural Lesion

- Control intracranial pressures.
- Elevate head to 30° to facilitate venous drainage from the intracranial vault.
- Consult neurosurgeon.

1.3 Intravenous Fluids

General Ref

- *Pediatrics* 2004;113:1279–1284
- *Pediatr Rev* 1993;14:70–79
- *Pediatr Rev* 2001;22:380
- *Pediatr Rev* 2002;23:371
- *Pediatrics* 2008;122:831–835

Def

- Current Segar and Holliday 100/50/20 (4/2/1) rule of maintenance volume estimates is based on the first 10/second 10/remaining kilograms of weight.
- Traditional use of ¼ NS for maintenance, ½ NS for replacement, and NS reserved for boluses has been implicated in evolution of hyponatremia in hospitalized pts.

Physiology

- Fluid needs related to size and metabolic rate.

- Approximately half of basal requirements are lost in urine output and half in "insensible losses."
- Pathologic states = extra losses occur via GI tract or into interstitial third space; healthy balanced state = approximately half daily fluid intake will be excreted by kidneys.
- From about age 3 yrs+, intracellular fluid comprises about 40% of body mass, with extracellular fluid about 20% (plasma volume: 5–8%); obesity lowers these percentages.

Complications

- Possible concern that traditional calculations can contribute to significant hyponatremia.
- Addition of potassium to fluids occurs after bolus completion; based on electrolyte levels and clinical situation.
- If renal shutdown is anticipated, waiting for renal flow establishment is cautious course.
- If normal potassium levels, add 20 mEq/L to meet maintenance and replacement needs. If low (3–3.5 mg%), then 30 mEq/L; if very low (< 3) then 40 mEq/L—all with follow-up monitoring.
- pH changes affect measured levels, with correction of acidosis leading to drops in extracellular K from shifts to the intracellular space (most pronounced in the correction of DKA). Thus, if pt is acidotic, increase potassium in the fluid.

Estimating Dehydration

- "% dehydration" is percentage of body weight lost as water.
  - Look for signs (check cap refill, turgor, mental status, mucous membranes, eyes, fontanelle, pulses). If positive signs, pt is likely at 5%.
  - If signs are striking before start of focused exam, pt likely at 10%.
  - If pt shows ashen color, weak pulses, delayed refill, lethargy, then likely approaching 15%.

- Decreased BP (by pediatric advanced life support definition) defines decompensated shock and requires *immediate* intervention (bone marrow needle if IV access difficult).
- Typical bolus is about 2% of body weight.
  - If in ballpark regarding estimates of maintenance, replacement, and losses, the child's homeostatic mechanisms will compensate for rest.
  - The sicker the pt, the more electrolyte monitoring is appropriate.

Hyponatremia

- Goal of hyponatremic dehydration correction is slow rise in sodium (Na) during rehydration.
- Sx such as seizures or altered mental status indicate use of 3% saline.
- Calculations assume the volume of distribution of sodium is approximately 0.6 body wt, and goal of correction is Na = 125.
- Example: A 10-kg child has Na 115; dose is 0.6 L/kg × 10 kg × 10 mEq/L = 60 mEq; 3% saline has approximately 1 mEq Na per 2 mL, so dose is 120 mL.
- A simple formula to remember is 12 mL/kg raises serum sodium by 10.
- If the child is hyponatremic but not symptomatic, use NS.
  - If hyponatremia is due to free water overload or syndrome of inappropriate [secretion of] antidiuretic hormone (as opposed to dehydration), treatment is fluid restriction.
  - Rare causes (require special intervention): kidney disease, adrenal insufficiency, undiagnosed CF, psychogenic polydipsia, cirrhosis and ascites, furosemide.
  - Serum Na may be low in the face of normal serum osmolarity with hyperlipidemia or hyperglycemia.
  - Formula for correction of glucose is division by 18 and for BUN, 2.8.

Hypernatremia: Now Rare

- Can occur from inappropriate formula mixing (not diluting concentrate), DI, or, rarely, from gastroenteritis.
- In the hyperosmolar state, perfusion and extracellular fluid volume are maintained at the expense of intracellular fluid.
- Finberg's correction fluid is adding an amp of calcium (Ca) gluconate to a liter of D5 ¼ NS with 40 mEq potassium chloride. This fluid avoids presenting hypotonic fluid to the CNS abruptly by using alternative cations to Na.
- Assume pt is 10% dehydrated and correct over 48 hr.
- Empirically, the children with hypernatremia are often Ca and K depleted and need these supplemented.

1.4   Diabetic Ketoacidosis

General Ref

- NICE guidelines 2002
- *Pediatrics* 2004;113:e133
- *Diabetes Care* 2006;29:1150

Cause

- Presenting feature of DM type 1.

Epidem

- Incidence 1–10%; 25% new-onset DM present with DKA.

S+S

- Polydipsia, polyuria, deep sighing, acidotic respiration, fruity breath, dehydration, drowsiness, abdominal pain/vomiting

Lab

- CBC, blood glucose, urea and electrolytes, including calcium, phosphate, and magnesium.
- ABGs; a raised amylase is common in DKA.
- Other investigations as indicated:
  - Chest Xray, CSF, throat swab, blood culture, UA, c + s

Complications

- Aspiration pneumonia (avoid by nasogastric tube if vomiting or impaired consciousness).
- Continuing abdominal pain is common and may be due to liver swelling, gastritis, bladder retention, or ileus.
- Cerebral edema leading to coma with 90% mortality 6–10 hr after starting treatment, especially in children with low pCO_2 and high BUN (*NEJM* 1985;312:1147).

Rx

- Monitoring of vital signs once per hr
- Strict input and output measurements
- Blood gases, electrolytes, glucose, calcium, phosphate, and magnesium q2–4h
- CBC, metabolic panel q6–8h
- Urine ketones until cleared

Strict Fluid Balance

- 10–20 mL/kg NS (0.9% NS) over 1–2 hr; repeat as needed.
- Rate of IV fluids for correction over 48 hr.
- First 4–6 hr: 0.9% NS then ½ NS.
- Add dextrose to IV fluids once BGL < 300 mg/dL.

Insulin

- 0.1 unit/kg per hr maintained to switch off ketogenesis.
- Once the pH > 7.3, consider reducing the insulin infusion rate to 0.05 units/kg per hr.
- Once pH maintained > 7.3 and pt is able to eat, may transition to sc insulin (ketones may not have disappeared completely before changing to sc insulin).
- Discontinue the insulin infusion 60 min (if using soluble or long-acting insulin) or 10 min (if using NovoRapid or Humalog) after the first sc injection to avoid rebound hyperglycemia.

1.5 Status Asthmaticus

General Ref

- *Am J Respir Crit Care Med* 2003;168:740
- *Chest* 2001;119:1913
- *Pediatr Drugs* 2001;3:509

Cause

- Worsening asthma refractory to treatment

Epidem

- Common PICU diagnosis

Pathophys

- Severe bronchospasms, inflammation, and edema of the airways; excess mucus production

S+S

- Unable to complete a sentence or too breathless to talk or feed.
- The following are life-threatening signs: hypotension, exhaustion, confusion, coma, a silent chest, cyanosis, poor respiratory effort.

Imaging

- Daily chest Xray in ventilated pts

Rx

- Urgent PICU admission.
- Continuous monitoring of heart rate, blood pressure, oxygen saturations, ABGs.
- High-flow humidified oxygen.
- Nebulized β-agonists, intermittently (2.5 mg albuterol or 5–10 mg terbutaline) or continuously (0.5 mg/kg per hr albuterol to a maximum of 20 mg/hr) with continuous monitoring for tachycardia and ventricular ectopy.
- Consider sc epinephrine or terbutaline if poor inspiratory effort compromises successful nebulizer treatment.
- Give systemic corticosteroids early in hx of severe asthma: IV 1 mg/kg methylprednisolone q6h.
- If symptoms refractory to initial β2 agonists, add inhaled anticholinergics: ipratropium bromide 250–500 μg/dose, mixed with β2 agonist.
- Consider IV β-agonists if no response to inhaled β-agonists (e.g., terbutaline 10 μg/kg loading dose followed by 0.5–5 μg/kg per min).
- Theophylline controversial; mixed results re benefit. Consider if unresponsive to maximal doses of bronchodilators and steroids.
- Magnesium sulphate ($MgSO_4$) effective in adults. Consider if worsening respiratory failure despite above 25–50 mg/kg per dose IV $MgSO_4$.
- If all of above fail, mechanical ventilation may be necessary; however, the goal should be to avoid because most of the morbidity occurring in asthma management is secondary to complications of ventilation.

Chapter 2

Neonatology

2.1 Neonatal Resuscitation

General Ref

- *Neonatal Resuscitation Program Manual*

Def

- Techniques used to expedite the adaptation of the newborn from the intrauterine environment to the extrauterine environment

Pathophys

- Likely necessary for infants experiencing respiratory distress syndrome (RDS) (hyaline membrane disease).
- More common for premature infants with immature lungs/respiratory processes.
- Without alveolar ventilation after birth, pulmonary circulation does not open up.
- In normal situations, it takes about 10 min for the healthy neonate to get to 95% saturation.

Interventions

- Concern over need for oxygen (O_2) in neonatal resuscitation due to possible production of reactive metabolites that can lead to cell damage.

- Hyperoxia also linked to chronic lung disease.
- Recent concern: possible association of hyperoxia with poor neurologic outcome, especially in tandem with hypocarbia.

Guidelines

- NRP recommends 100% O_2 for initial resuscitation.
- Saturations in premature infants (especially < 32 weeks of gestation where retina is vulnerable): target in low 90s.
- Meconium-stained fluid:
  - Now thought to be marker for asphyxia in selected cases.
  - Generally, meconium is *not* in the airway, only in the gi tract.
  - Resuscitate as if no meconium present unless infant shows sx of in utero aspiration (typically depressed, asphyxiated, postmature, dysmature neonates).

Physical Exam

- Heart rate (HR) and respiratory effectiveness are linked.
- Initiate bag-valve-mask device to start ventilation if respiration not spontaneous or if HR remains < 100 bpm (see NRP guidelines).
- Intubation not necessary immediately unless anatomic variant in airway, or if extremely low birthweight infant with inability to get mask to seal well.
- Effective ventilation leads to chest movement, breath sounds, and rise in HR.

2.2 Sepsis

General Ref

- *N Engl J Med* 347:240
- *Pediatrics* 1999;103:e360
- Avery's *Diseases of the Newborn*, 8th ed., Chap 39
- *Arch Dis Child* 2009;163:6–13

Def

- Multisystem impairment along with a positive bacterial culture from a usually sterile site.
- May have negative culture but treated on the basis of clinical findings and suspicious laboratory markers.
- Si + sx of sepsis are inconsistent (especially early) and overlap with other serious and less serious neonatal conditions.

Epidem

- Estimated 600,000 newborns evaluated for sepsis annually; one-third to three-quarters are subsequently exposed to antibiotics.
- Risk factors for bacterial infection include prematurity, prolonged rupture of membranes, maternal chorioamnionitis, group B strep (GBS) colonization (also low APGAR scores and male sex: reason unknown).
- Incidence of true sepsis is thought to be declining with GBS prophylaxis.
- More than 50% of sepsis cases do *not* involve GBS.

Clinical Findings

- Are all nonspecific, and each has its own differential diagnosis.
- Presenting or associated sx: fever (approximately 50%), hypothermia (15%), respiratory distress (33%), apnea (22%), cyanosis (24%), vomiting (25%) abdomen distention (17%), vomiting or anorexia (25%).
- Physical findings include tachycardia, poor perfusion, hepatomegaly, or jaundice.

Lab

- Band count > 2000, immature neutrophil to total neutrophil ratio > 0.2, total neutrophil number > 1750, or total WBC < 5000.

- Can add an acute phase reactant, such as the CRP, to add specificity.
- Vast majority of infants treated with antibiotics are not septic (defined as positive culture) due to high sensitivity of lab tests.
- Blood counts and acute phase reactants are typically used to define infants with "sepsis suspected, not proven."
- If serial lab values are normal when rechecked at 12 and 36 hr of life, can stop treatment when blood culture is returned negative.
- New test for "universal primer PCR" relies on finding segments of the 16S ribosomal RNA common to all bacteria (but not found in other organisms). When *no* antibiotics are on board, this test looks to be more sensitive and specific (both in high 90s) than other lab tests.

Rx

- Culture (blood: minimum 1 mL for accuracy) and start on antibiotics pending results.
- If serial labs not reassuring despite improved clinical findings, continue treatment for 1 wk.
- If blood culture is positive, extend rx to 10 d.
- Antibiotic recommendations: ampicillin 100 mg/kg initially, then 50 mg/kg q8h (to cover Listeria and GBS) with gentamicin once daily dosing at 4 mg/kg in term infants (2.5/kg q12h for premature infants) for extended gram-negative coverage.
- If CSF is abnormal, cefotaxime is added (better CNS penetration).
- Severely compromised infants need cardiopulmonary support, NBICU, IV fluids for glucose support until well enough to feed, close monitoring for apnea.
- Group B strep:
  - Currently the major pathogen involved in early-onset sepsis.
  - Web site http://www.cdc.gov/groupbstrep/hospitals/hospitals_guidelines.htm presents the most recent guidelines for management of both mother and newborn.

- Algorithm for neonates involves observation for 48 hr after birth for all exposed infants, unless ideal conditions are met: maternal treatment 4 hr or more, 38 wk or more of gestation, reliable family, no sx.

2.3 Newborn Discharge Exam

General Ref
- Goldenring, *Contemp Pediatr*, April 1, 2007
- *Pediatr Rev* 2006;27:89–98

Def
- Routine postpartum stay guidelines include genetic and hearing screening, monitoring for hyperbilirubinemia, surveillance for GBS complications.
- Specific high-risk situations may require extra monitoring [blood glucose for large gestational age (LGA) infants or infants of diabetic mother (IDM), minimal length of stay for late-preterm infants, etc.].
- Checklist for discharge should include the following:
  - Lactation consultation: effective latch, adequate milk supply (or stimulation of milk supply), establishment of feeding plan. In difficult situations, suggest home pumping or syringe feeding. All breastfeeding babies need 48-hr postdischarge follow-up (home visit, office, hospital nursery) for feeding assessment and wt check. Frequency of voids and stools, serial weights, and observation of nursing pattern are synthesized to gauge necessity of intervention.
  - Vitamin supplementation: vitamin D for breastfed babies (new recommendations, 2008 AAP); iron supplementation required at 6 months.

NEONATOLOGY

- Tobacco smoke exposure: caution about effects of environmental tobacco smoke if household members smoke.
- Jaundice assessment (AAP guidelines): discuss risk status and monitoring at discharge.
- Sleep safety: "back to sleep" until 6 months. No heavy blankets, beanbag or extra-soft cushion mattresses; co-sleeping increases sudden infant death syndrome (SIDS) risk; don't overheat.
- Home safety: smoke alarms, fire escape routes planned.
- Toxin awareness: pesticides, household sprays/cleansers, potential lead hazards.
- Outdoor safety: car seats, cold exposure (winter), sun and insect protection (summer).
- Routine care: baby skin, diaper rashes, cord care, filing nails, circumcision or foreskin care, vaginal cleansing.
- Normal gi patterns: spitting, diarrhea, constipation.
- Crying: normal patterns in babies. Reinforce: *never shake a baby*.
- Infant illness assessment: taking a temperature, assessing alertness, assessing breathing.
- Postpartum depression: available resources.
- How to contact pediatric office/follow-up care, importance of immunizations, hepatitis B at discharge.
- Suggest family members be immunized against pertussis and influenza.
- Obtain detailed hx of genetic/familial conditions at discharge or 2-wk follow-up.

2.4 Meconium Aspiration Syndrome

General Ref

- Wiswell et al, *Pediatrics* 2000;105:1–7
- Dargaville et al, *Pediatrics* 2006;117:1712–1721

Def

- Newborn respiratory distress associated with in utero aspiration of meconium mixed with amniotic fluid

Pathophys

- Meconium aspiration syndrome (MAS) is intertwined with neonatal asphyxia and fetal distress.
- Meconium particulate matter can act like a ball valve; pneumothorax is frequent complication.
- Bile salts and other components lead to irritative pneumonitis.
- Meconium interferes with surfactant function, so alveolar function becomes increasingly unstable.

Epidem

- Meconium fluid observed in approximately 12% of term births (less frequent with preterms), but only 2% have complications.
- Typically a postmature, dysmature infant manifesting fetal distress on the monitor, low APGAR at 5 min, requiring resuscitation in the delivery room.
- Less commonly, infant emerge with spontaneous cry but develop signs of distress in first hours of life. The latter group generally develops only mild disease but occasionally can get complications of air leak, pulmonary hypertension, and so on, needing aggressive management.

Management

- Most infants have no pulmonary symptoms; therefore aggressive airway intervention is not only unnecessary, but potentially harmful.
- Tracheal suctioning prior to positive pressure is recommended for the depressed newborn (re: removal of some aspirated material might modify disease course).

Complications/Rx

- Infants with the full MAS require NBICU management with assisted ventilation; monitor for air leaks, fluid and glucose support.
- In severe cases, high-frequency ventilation, nitric oxide, or extracorporeal membrane oxygenation (ECMO) becomes necessary to treat profound hypoxemia.
- Empirical antibiotics typically are part of regimen, pending cultures.
- Neurologic monitoring for effects of associated perinatal asphyxia is also necessary.

2.5   Transient Tachypnea of the Newborn

General Ref

- *Pediatr Rev* 1995;16:209–217
- *Pediatr Rev* 2008;29:e59–e65

Def

- Generally transient tachypnea of the newborn (TTN) is a self-limited condition, thought to be related to disruption of fetal lung fluid resorption, leading to varying levels of respiratory distress and hypoxemia in the first hr(s) to days of life.

Diff Dx

- RDS, air leaks, MAS, sepsis, withdrawal, metabolic derangements: these conditions need more aggressive respiratory interventions as well as specific management of the underlying condition.
- TTN often is a diagnosis of exclusion.

Epidem

- Approximately 5 in 1000 births overall; more common after caesarean deliveries, especially if it occurs in absence of labor (alteration of epinephrine dynamics affect both sodium pumps and lymphatic flow).
- Other risk factors: IDM, macrosomia, late preterm, male sex.
- Theoretically, TTN might be a manifestation of genetically transmitted tendency to lung dysfunction.

Clinical

- Typical case presents in the first minutes to hours with grunting, flaring, retractions, and tachypnea.
- Hypoxemia is variable, but unusual to require more than 40% O_2 to maintain saturations in the 90s.
- Duration of symptoms that defines TTN versus "delayed transition": approximately 6 hr. Most infants resolve in first 24 hr, but some persist with increased respiratory rate (RR) and low-grade O_2 requirement for 72+ hr.

Lab

- Chest Xray shows perihilar streaking, hyperinflation, fluid in the interlobar fissures.
- Can have fluffy infiltrates that obscure the heart border or diaphragm.
- Film used to rule out air leaks, surgical lung diseases, pneumonia, and RDS.
- More challenging cases with higher O_2 requirements and RR often need NBICU for monitoring as well as specialty help to rule out alternative diagnoses.

Treatment

- Supportive:
  - O_2 to keep saturation in the low 90s; IV fluids to maintain normal range blood sugar.

- Many of these infants are on antibiotics for variable period of time pending the results of sepsis workup, serial CBCs, acute phase reactants.
- In premature infants, difficult to separate from infant respiratory distress syndrome or infection
- Infants often worked up for early-onset sepsis and put on antibiotic therapy pending serial blood counts, acute phase reactants, and culture results

Complications

- Occur more from unrecognized alternative dx than from TTN: untreated sepsis, unrecognized congenital heart disease.
- In rare situations, what's thought to be TTN is complicated by an air leak or, very rarely, persistent pulmonary hypertension of newborn (PPHN).

Prevention

- Minimizing late preterm deliveries may be challenging when they are related to spontaneous onset of labor.
- Plan elective caesarean deliveries beyond 39 weeks for prevention.

2.6 Neonatal Hypoglycemia

General Ref

- Cornblath, *Pediatrics* 2000;105:1141

Def

- Normal blood sugar is ≥ 45 or more the first day of life and ≥ 50 thereafter.
- Unfortunately, exact level that puts infants at neurodevelopmental risk is not known and likely varies.

Pathophys

- Typically a combination of inadequate substrate or hyperinsulinism.
- Classic situation is a macrosomic IDM; infant will need parenteral glucose support until pancreas adjusts to extrauterine environment.
- Other possibility is small for gestational age (SGA) infant or late preterm, where liver glycogen stores may be limited; need early and frequent feeding to keep glucose levels in the normal range; IV if respiratory issues make po or ng route impossible.
- Rare: insulin-secreting tumors, nesidioblastosis, or inborn errors of metabolism.

Lab

- Blood glucose from lab to confirm low levels.
- Whole blood levels are 15% lower than plasma and are even lower if polycythemia.
- Levels also will fall if the blood is not run fresh.
- Who to screen:
  - Infant > 4 kg or < 2 kg; LGA or SGA (using 90th and 10th percentiles for gestation).
  - IDM (including gestation ≤ 37 wks), suspected sepsis, significant perinatal distress or APGAR > 5 at 5 min, mother on terbutaline or β-blocker, stigmata of Beckwith's, polycythemia, congenital heart disease.
  - Avoid screening "normal" newborns; they often have borderline values of unclear significance.
  - Screen IDMs soon after birth and hourly for 3 d (assuming normal).
  - Screen other categories at 1 hr and every 2 hr for 3 d. Levels obtained determine further testing and interventions.

Sx

- Typically asymptomatic.
- Hypoglycemia can cause jitteriness, apnea, hypotonia, altered consciousness, poor feeding, seizures, tachypnea. Test for low blood sugar if infant is symptomatic and proceed with aggressive management.

Rx

- Asymptomatic infants can be given oral substrate and rechecked.
- If feedings unsuccessful, IV dextrose is indicated.
- Begin IV therapy with "mini bolus" of 2–3 mL/kg D10W over a few min, followed by IV D10 at 5 mL/kg per hr, with goal to achieve a level of 50.
- Monitor response and increase dextrose concentration to 12.5% if necessary.
- Next step is hydrocortisone in consultation with a neonatal center.
- If the infant responds to feeds, check levels until 2–3 are normal and feeds are established.
- Prolonged hypoglycemia:
  - Majority resolve by 2–3 d of age.
  - Persistent findings suggest possibility of endocrinopathy or inborn error.
  - If persistent low blood sugar, draw blood for cortisol, growth hormone, insulin, and urine ketones.

2.7   Unconjugated Hyperbilirubinemia

General Ref

- Newman et al, *N Engl J Med* 2006;354:1889–1900
- Maisels, *N Engl J Med* 2008;358:920–928
- Guidelines, *Pediatrics* 2004;114:297–316

Def

- Elevation of total bilirubin (minus "direct" component).
- At extreme levels can lead to diffusion of free bilirubin through blood-brain barrier and neurologic sequelae.
- Monitoring and management to prevent kernicterus.
- Total bilirubin (TB) is measured serially; cannot accurately estimate free bilirubin due to tight binding to albumen.

Pathophys

- TB level universally elevated in infants postnatally due to normal physiology.
- Processes that lead to increased load of bilirubin precursors, slow down hepatic transferases, or increase enterohepatic circulation can affect the duration and peak level of jaundice.
- "Normal" peak is < 12; occurs between 3rd and 5th day of life.
- 7–8% of infants > 12, but < 2% reach 20.
- Kernicterus is extremely rare in otherwise healthy infants < 30.
- Increased risk of kernicterus due to hemolytic processes (particularly G6PD deficiency), diseases that affect bilirubin binding (sepsis, acidosis), or breach the blood-brain barrier (intracranial bleeding).
- Presence of "direct" jaundice is indicative of hepatic pathology.

Dx

- Bilirubin level defines the degree of concern. AAP guidelines stratify infants into different risk categories for follow-up need, based on bilirubin level, age in hours, comorbid illnesses, gestation, and so on.
- Guidelines also set the level at which phototherapy or exchange transfusion should be instituted, again based on bilirubin level, age in hr, and comorbidities.

- Blood type and direct Coombs test rule out significant immunohemolysis.
- CBC for anemia; smear for RBC morphology (check for hemolysis).
- Infants may be rehospitalized if encounter lactation delay postdischarge.
- Serum sodium to assess for associated electrolyte disturbances.
- Serial wt and careful hx assessing suck and swallow; voids and stools for dx.

Rx

- 2004 AAP guidelines are current standard of care.
- Intensive phototherapy as described in the AAP guidelines leads to the most rapid decline; supply eye protection to infant if under light sources shining down.
- Establish feeding plan to rehydrate infant (consider IV fluids), decrease enterohepatic circulation, and promote lactation success.

Prognosis

- The main goal of any postdischarge monitoring program should be to prevent extreme levels.
- Kernicteric levels can occur in otherwise healthy infants with just exaggerated "physiologic" jaundice from some combination of genetic predisposition and feeding/enterohepatic issues.
- AAP recommends obtaining a level on all infants at discharge and establishing degree of risk through their nomogram; all infants should be assessed postdischarge at 3–5 d of age: Check bilirubin if suspect jaundice clinically.
- Epidemiologic risk factors for kernicterus include "late pre-term" infants, South Asian background, male, breastfeeding.
- Babies with jaundice noted in first 24 hr are likely to have some hemolytic pathology, although more likely to be identified.

2.8   Conjugated Hyperbilirubinemia

Def

- Elevations of conjugated bilirubin > 2 mg% or > 20% of total bilirubin.
- Labs sometimes measure conjugated bilirubin and "delta bilirubin" (conjugated bilirubin attached to albumen) together when reporting "direct" fraction. Delta bilirubin can last for weeks in serum and give false impression of persistent disease. Ask lab to separate out if values are not making sense.

Normal Phys

- Albumen-bound bilirubin separated from carrier and incorporated into hepatocyte by membrane carrier protein.
- Bilirubin carried by glutathione-S-transferase to endoplasmic reticulum where it is conjugated by UGT1A1 enzyme into monoand diglucuronides.
- Specialized transport proteins remove conjugated bilirubin from the hepatocytes and carry it to the bile canaliculi for excretion.

Pathophys

- Usual neonatal jaundice is unconjugated and there is no hepatocellular disease; babies have orange, as opposed to greenish, hue.
- Liver disease produces mixed hyperbilirubinemia because both conjugation and excretion are disordered.
- Some rare defects in the normal excretion transport pathway can lead to conjugated jaundice (Dubin-Johnson, Rotor's, etc.).
- In neonates, r/o extrahepatic biliary atresia because outcome of a Kasai procedure depends on timely diagnosis.

Causes in Neonates

- Rule out extrahepatic biliary atresia.
- Idiopathic neonatal hepatitis (histologic diagnosis on biopsy); α-1 AT deficiency; Alagille's syndrome (dysmorphic, often have cardiac findings); viral infections (toxoplasmosis, other infections, rubella, cytomegalovirus, and herpes simplex, hepatitis B, HIV, other); bacterial infections (sepsis, UTI, necrotizing enterocolitis); toxic exposure; CF, thyroid (usually unconjugated); lipid storage diseases; amino acid disorders; galactosemia; glycogen storage disorders.
- Imaging for choledochal cyst, vascular tumors, or other mass for surgical removal.
- Radionucleotide scans to trace excretion into the gi tract.
- Follow lab studies and imaging with biopsy for definitive dx.
- Refer to pediatric center with gi and surgery.

Causes in Older Children

- Acute onset typically from hepatitis A or Epstein-Barr virus, although a variety of other viruses and HIV can be involved; consider toxic exposures and medications.
- R/o Wilson's disease in chronic cases; copper studies (decreased ceruloplasmin; increased urinary copper) can be useful.
- Autoimmune hepatitis usually associated with immune markers (ANA/anti SMA or anti LKM1).
- Some conditions appear with clinical liver dysfunction, such as CF, α-1AT, Alagille's, hypothyroid.
- Consider hemochromatosis, parasites, choledochal cysts and other surgical lesions, and gallstones/sludging (more common in older children).
- May need bx for definitive dx.

2.9 Cyanotic Newborn

General Ref

- Osborn, *Pediatrics*, Chap. 203, "Disorders of the Cardiovascular System of the Newborn"
- *Pediatr Rev* 2009;30:2, "Pulmonary Hypertension"

Def

- An infant who remains cyanotic (and *usually* desaturated) despite O_2 therapy.
- It takes about 3 g% desaturated hgb for a white person to look cyanotic, and fetal hgb has its dissociation curve shifted to the left.
- At any given PO_2 saturation, an infant will have a *higher* saturation than an adult and look *less* cyanotic; visible cyanosis in a newborn correlates with a saturation > 80–85%, varying with hgb.

Diff Dx

- Consider whether heart disease, lung disease, or hgb abnormality is causing cyanosis.
- PPHN usually is associated with some element of lung parenchymal disease, with the degree of hypoxia out of proportion to the amount of lung injury. Although it is technically "lung disease," there is right-left shunting analogous to cardiac disease, in this case predominantly "backward" through the ductus (or through the foramen ovale).

Epidem

- Overall incidence of cyanotic lesions in newborns is rare, approximately 1 in 2000; cyanosis in conjunction with lung disease in PPHN is estimated at 2 in 1000 term births.

Pathophys

- Impaired diffusion and O_2 transfer underlies most common causes of cyanosis, such as TTN, pneumonia, or RDS in premature infants.
- Possible intrapulmonary physiologic shunting from ventilation perfusion ratio mismatch, although usually responsive delivering high concentrations of O_2.
- Likewise, with peripheral cyanosis due to poor perfusion, arterial saturations will be normal with the cyanosis due to increased extraction at the tissue level.
- Right-left shunting does not respond to O_2 (see later).

Physical Exam

- Assess breathing to determine if lung disease is primary or secondary.
- Perform cardiac exam to look for signs of cyanotic heart disease; may hear a click (truncus), loud single second heart sound (transposition of the great arteries), systolic murmur (tetralogy, tricuspid atresia), hepatomegaly (total anomalous pulmonary venous return); definitive dx depends on echocardiogram (ECHO) findings.

Lab

- O_2 saturations not sensitive enough; therefore ABGs are necessary. Correlative ABGs would show a PaO_2 difference of 20 mm Hg.
- Recommend *hyperoxia test* for underlying cause; a PaO_2 rise to > 150 would be unusual in the presence of right-left shunting. Elevated PCO_2 also suggests lung disease.
- If ABG testing not feasible, then a preductal saturation to 99% on 100% O_2 correlates somewhat.

Imaging

- Chest Xrays (lung disease, cardiac anatomy); EKG (heart lesions); ECHO (if cardiologist on site)

Methemoglobinemia

- Rare disorder of hgb metabolism where the ferric (oxidized) state of iron is not recirculated to the ferrous state and the molecule is unable to bind O_2. Circulatory and clinical effects are analogous to anemia. Dx via drawing "chocolate"-colored venous blood and watch that it does not turn pink on exposure to air. Typically, O_2 saturation will be low, but PO_2 on ABG measurement will be normal in room air and elevated in O_2.

2.10   Newborn Metabolic Screen

General Ref

- *Pediatrics* 2008;121:193–217
- http://genes-r-us.uthscsa.edu

Def

- All US-born infants are offered some degree of newborn metabolic screening through filter paper blood drop analysis.
- Document results in infant's record, but remember these tests are not 100% sensitive and hx of in-range screening results does not eliminate the possibility that a symptomatic child has one of the covered conditions.

History

- Screens generally look for phenylketonuria (PKU), galactosemia, maple syrup urine disease (MSUD), homocystinuria, hypothyroidism, biotinidase deficiency, CAH, hemoglobinopathies, and CF screening.
- Some states collect a second sample at 1–2 wk of age for greater sensitivity.

Pathophys

- The classic inborn errors are related to enzyme defects that block a specific pathway, typically leading to the accumulation of a toxic metabolite, as in PKU, or a deficiency of the end product, as in CAH. Biotinidase deficiency is unique in that it relates to a defect in vitamin recycling. Most congenital hypothyroidism is from aplasia of the gland itself.
- Clinical outcomes range from silent brain injury (PKU, thyroid) to acute metabolic emergency (MSUD, CAH, and galactosemia); screening is used to guide intervention.

Dx

- Contact genetics/metabolism experts to assist with initial management and follow-up.
- See American College of Medical Genetics Web site (www .acmg.net) for links to ACTion sheets that cover all "abnormal" screens and algorithms for guidance on further testing to confirm dx.

Management

- Abnormal results fall into three categories along with identification of cases: false positives, carrier state identification, and true indeterminates. Employ the assistance of a genetics specialist when counseling families.
- Screen siblings of identified pts; some may have disease, others may be carriers.

2.11 Hearing Screen

General Ref

- *Pediatr Rev* 2009;30:207–215
- *N Engl J Med* 2000;342:1101–1109

- *Pediatrics* 2008;121:1119–1126
- *Pediatrics* 2006;117;e631–e636
- US Preventive Services Task Force (USPSTF), *Pediatrics* 2008;122:1

Def

- Universal newborn screening for hearing loss has become standard of care in most states based on the concept of "critical periods" for neurodevelopment.
- Risk factors are identifiable in < 50% of infants found with true loss.
- The USPSTF gives Universal Newborn Hearing Screening (UNHS) a B rating.

Epidem

- Projected incidence of 1–3 per 1000 births

Pathophys

- Hearing loss can be subdivided into sensorineural hearing loss (SNHL) (defect in the neurology of the hearing apparatus), conductive hearing loss (interference with the transmission of sound waves to the nerves), and central hearing loss (deficiency in neural processing from the brainstem to cortical centers). UNHS focuses on SNHL.
- In utero infections may or may not have been obvious; other risk factors include exposure to ototoxic drugs, hypoxic-ischemic encephalopathy, extreme prematurity, extreme hyperbilirubinemia.

Universal Screening Methodology

- Screening to assess either OAE (otoacoustic emissions) or ABR (auditory brainstem response).
- OAE assumes a healthy cochlea emits signals in response to clicks; a "failed" response can be repeated hours later to achieve a "pass," avoiding referral.

NEONATOLOGY

- 90% of persistent failures pass on follow-up, usually with ABR device.
- ABR screens measures EEG waveforms in response to clicks.
- State programs attempt to confirm or pass all positive screens by 1 month of age, requiring assistance from primary care to help with the logistics of follow-up. Persistent failed screens leads to more complex ABR testing that estimates degree of impairment, as well as ENT evaluation to rule out anatomic abnormalities, followed by assessment for amplification.
- Goal is to provide intervention for true positives by 3–6 months.

Later Onset Sensorineural Hearing Loss

- Accounted for about 25% of children with persistent hearing deficiency in a population study from Austria (*Pediatrics* 2006;117)
- Causes included cytomegalovirus, meningitis, syndromes, family hx, exposure to ototoxic drugs, serious illness requiring ECMO. Thus, children with risk factors or clinical findings do need periodic assessment.

Hearing Screening in Older Children

- Up until age 4–6 yr, hearing screening requires an audiologist with specialized equipment; later, conventional audiometry with earphones is available at most primary care offices.
- "Visual reinforcement audiometry" is useful from about 9–30 months; the equipment is normed for frequency-specific thresholds by age.
- "Play audiometry" is applied to children from 30 months of age to school age and can measure bone as well as air thresholds.

Decibel Scale

- Logarithmic, so 20 dB sound has 10 times the physical power of 10 dB.

- Cutoffs for hearing impairment: normal < 15; minimal < 25; moderate < 55; moderate to severe < 70; severe < 90; profound 90+.
- Speech reception requires acuity in the 1000–2000 Hz frequency range, and at the "moderate" range of impairment (25–55 dB) 50–100% of normal volume speech may be missed.

2.12   Brachial Plexus Injury

General Ref

- Lovell and Winter's *Pediatric Orthopedics*, 6th ed., pp. 926–932
- Piatt, *Pediatr Clin North Am* 2004;51:421–440
- Joyner and Soto, *Pediatr Rev* 2006;27:238–239

Def

- Spectrum of problems relating to intrapartum injury to the complex set of lower cervical and upper thoracic nerves (C5 through T1).
- Typical causes: traction on the head along with extreme lateral flexion during a difficult delivery (macrosomia from IDM, shoulder dystocia, abnormal lie); intrauterine pressure on the shoulder against the sacrum.
- Speed of recovery or permanence of injury relates to degree of damage to the nerves.

Epidem

- 1 in 1000 live births.
- Most common type is Erb's palsy involving the upper nerve roots C5-C7.
- On exam, the biceps reflex will be absent, Moro asymmetric, but grasp present.

Lab Studies

- Xrays of clavicle and humerus for associated fractures.
- Chest Xray to document diaphragmatic motion because ipsilateral phrenic nerve damage in lower plexus injury (T1) can cause lack of function.
- Eye exam for Horner's syndrome (miosis, ptosis).

Management

- Immobilization of the affected arm for first 10–14 d (longer if humerus fractured); referral to physical therapist after immobilization period.
- If no improvement, refer to specialty center.
- Surgical judgment needed if early progress, but unsatisfactory residual function at 6–12 months.

Prognosis

- Successful spontaneous recovery usually begins early; Erb's has best outcome (90% recover without major intervention).
- Lower plexus and total plexus injuries are more likely to be permanent.
- Of the pts that show improvement by 3 months, function may continue to improve over first 12–18 months.

Complications

- Traction on the nerves can be transmitted centrally to the cord and lead to a "pseudosyrinx" on imaging; generally asymptomatic and nonprogressive.
- Orthopedic deformities of the shoulder joint can complicate prolonged muscle imbalance, leading to deficient molding of the "socket" (glenoid dysplasia) and in more severe cases actual posterior dislocation of the humerus; requires complex pediatric orthopedic interventions.

2.13   Developmental Dysplasia of the Hip

General Ref

- *Pediatrics* 2006;117:e557–e576
- *Pediatrics* 2000;105:896–905

Def

- Developmental dysplasia of the hip (DDH) reflects the understanding that the hip may not be "out" at birth but dislocates later due to disruption of the normal process of acetabular development.
- Screening to prevent long-term disability from premature degenerative joint disease and chronic pain.

Epidem

- Incidence range is 1.5–20 per 1000 births; in United States, approximately 11.5 overall. Relative risk (RR) 4.6 in girls versus boys; RR 7.0 for breech; breech female incidence rate is 133 per 1000.
- Other risk factors: fetal constraint from LGA or oligohydramnios, lower limb deformities, ethnicity (Native American), positive family history.
- 75% of cases occur in absence of risk factors (except female).
- 60–80% of cases identified by physical exam in newborns resolve spontaneously by 2–8 wk; 90% of those with mild dysplasia resolve spontaneously between 6 wk and 6 months.

Pathophys

- Hormonally induced laxity of capsular structures may allow the femoral head to spontaneously move in and out of joint. Leg extension (as in cradle boarding) promotes dislocation; abduction inhibits (frog-leg, triple diapering).

Physical Exam

- Classic screening tests are Barlow and Ortolani maneuvers.
- Barlow (dislocation) test: infant's thigh is adducted with hips and knees flexed to 90°, apply gentle downward pressure in attempt to push femoral head out from the socket. Positive finding is a "clunk" as hip dislocates.
- Ortolani (relocation) maneuver: hold infant's thigh with the middle finger over the trochanter, first lifting up and then abducting the thigh with medial pressure exerted on the trochanter. Positive finding is a clunk as the hip relocates.

Radiology Findings

- AAP guidelines suggest ultrasound if any equivocal physical findings on exam or if baby was breech. Optimal time for study is 6 wk of age.

Rx

- Goal is to promote normal anatomic development by keeping femoral head in place. Most common technique is Pavlik harness.
- In situations where the hip cannot be relocated for splinting, traction may allow for subsequent closed reduction and casting.
- In severe cases, surgical reduction or even osteotomies are needed, with subsequent spica casting.
- Complications of therapy include usual anesthesia risk if surgery needed, skin breakdown, peripheral nerve injury.

2.14   Testicular Torsion

Cause

- Inadequate testicular fixation; leading to torsion of the cord structures, vascular compromise, and eventually infarction of gonadal tissue.

Epidem

- Can occur in utero or neonatal. Most in pubertal teenagers.

History

- Sudden onset severe testicular, groin, or lower abdominal pain. Often vomiting. Sometimes with exercise or minor trauma, can be during sleep. A third may have had previous transient pain episode (intermittent torsion).

Physical Exam

- Key finding is high riding testicle on painful side and *lack* of cremaster reflex. May be reactive hydrocele. Scrotum appears reddened, and a tender testicle may be lying horizontally.

Complications

- Loss of testicular viability: 98% salvage in first 6 hr, declining to 0–20% over the following 24 hr.

Diagnostic Test

- Doppler ultrasound. Torsion shows decreased flow.

Rx

- Urology referral. Occasionally manual reduction is successful, followed by elective orchiopexy. Usually immediate surgical reduction and repair is necessary.

Diff Dx

- Torsion of appendix testis more common in prepubertal. Cremaster maintained, and localized pain over upper pole with "blue dot" sign. Treated with time. Epididymitis common in all age ranges and has more subacute onset. Cremaster intact. Treated with antibiotics and consideration given to associated UTI or sexually transmitted disease. Rare causes of scrotal pain include Henoch-Schönlein purpura, viral orchitis, tumor, referred pain from abdominal pathology, even appendicitis.

2.15 Undescended Testes (Cryptorchidism)

Gen Ref
- *Pediatr Clin North Am* 1998;45:813–830
- *N Engl J Med* 2007;356:1835–1841

Cause
- Testes fail to complete proper descent and remain in abdominal cavity or palpable in the inguinal canal.

Epidem
- 2% of term babies have bilateral and 3% unilateral undescended testicles (UDTs). Incidence is higher in premature babies, because testicular descent into the inguinal canal only begins in the third trimester. By 3 months, overall rate is 1.5% with little change after that. Pathophysiology is not well understood.

S+S
- Bimanual testicular exam may differentiate retractile from UDTs.
- Look for features of an associated syndrome (most cases idiopathic).
- Note size, consistency, and compare position on two sides.
- Phenotypic males with bilateral UDTs need a workup to r/o congenital adrenal hyperplasia or an intersex disorder.

Complications
- Subfertility, inguinal hernia, testicular torsion, malignant change (orchiopexy does not affect malignant transformation) (*Cancer* 1982;49:1023–1030).

Lab

- Bilateral UDTs
- Electrolytes, LH, FSH, testosterone, adrenal hormones/metabolites
- Karyotype

Xray

- Pelvic ultrasound: to exclude a uterus and look for gonads

Rx

- Follow up and observe to 3 months; most will have descended by this time.
- If not descended, refer to surgery.
- Orchiopexy usually carried out at 1–2 yr to maximize fertility.

2.16   Inguinal Hernia

Gen Ref

- *J Pediatr Surg* 2006;41:1999
- *J Pediatr Surg* 2005;40:1163

Cause

- Almost always indirect in children; due to a patent process vaginalis

Epidem

- 1–5% of newborns; more common in premature babies
- 10% bilateral in full term and 50% in premature
- 4M:F; more common on the right in both sexes

S+S

- Intermittent swelling in the groin or scrotum with crying or straining

- May present as an irreducible, firm, tender, lump in the groin or scrotum

Lab

- Generally not helpful; no correlation between WBC and degree of vascular compromise in incarcerated hernias.
- Consider karyotyping if testes noted in inguinal canal.

Rx

- Surgery is the definitive management.
- If irreducible, manual reduction with analgesia should be attempted (successful in 95–100% of cases), followed by delayed elective surgery; fewer complications with this approach versus emergent surgery.
- Incarcerated hernia: Keep NPO if emergent surgical reduction of manual reduction fails.
- Surgery involves ligation and division of the process vaginalis via an inguinal skin crease incision.
- Good results are obtained with laparoscopic herniorrhaphy.
- Repair should occur promptly once diagnosed due to risk of strangulation.

2.17 Hydrocele

Gen Ref

- *Urol Clin North Am* 1995;22:119–130

Cause

- Collection of fluid along patent process vaginalis

S+S

- Asymptomatic, nontender, often bilateral, scrotal swelling.
- Swelling transilluminates.

Course

- Most resolve spontaneously.

Rx

- If no resolution by 18 months, surgery required

2.18 Hypospadias

Gen Ref

- *J Urol* 1999;162:1003–1006

Cause

- Failure of normal proximodistal urethral tubularization that occurs normally under the influence of testosterone; results in a urethral opening proximal to the normal meatus on the glans.
- More common if family hx

Epidem

- Common congenital anomaly; affects 1 in 200 boys. Studies suggest unexplained increasing incidence.

S+S

- Look for associated anomalies (e.g., hernia, cryptorchidism).
- Ventral urethral meatus, hooded dorsal foreskin (foreskin fails to fuse ventrally), and a chordee (ventral curvature of the penile shaft).
- Urethral opening may be glanular or coronal (most common types) or midshaft or penoscrotal.

Lab

- Karyotype if also bilateral UDTs.

Rx

- Circumcision is contraindicated because foreskin needed for reconstruction.
- Surgery: in 1st year of life (before 2 yr of age).

2.19   Circumcision

Gen Ref

- *Pediatrics* 1999;103:686–693
- *N Engl J Med* 2009;360:1298-1309

General

- Foreskin is adherent to the surface of the glans at birth.
- Avoid forced retraction.
- By 1 yr of age, 50% of boys have retractile foreskins, by 4 yr, 90%; and by 16 yr, 99%.
- Ballooning with micturition can occur if foreskin is nonretractile, which is physiologic.

Circumcision

- There are very few medical indications.
- AAP (American Academy of Pediatrics) Circumcision Policy Statement states that though there may be benefits to the procedure, there is insufficient evidence to recommend it should be done routinely (*Pediatrics* 1999; 103:686–693).

Medical Indications

- Phimosis:
  - Rare < 5 yr of age (normal nonretractile foreskin often misdiagnosed as phimosis)

- Due to balanitis xerotica obliterans, a skin condition that causes whitish scarring of foreskin and may cause urethral stenosis
- Recurrent balanoposthitis:
  - Inflammation of glans and foreskin in an uncircumcised male
  - Etiology multifactorial but typically due to poor hygiene in children
  - Redness and purulent discharge common
  - Rx: warm baths and broad-spectrum antibiotics with circumcision if attacks are recurrent

2.20 Cleft Lip and Palate

Cause

- Unilateral or bilateral
- Cleft lip: failure of fusion of the frontonasal and maxillary processes
- Cleft palate: failure of fusion of the palatine processes and the nasal septum
- Most polygenic inheritance but may be part of a syndrome
- Association with maternal anticonvulsant therapy

Epidem

- Affect 0.8 per 1000 infants; third most common congenital anomaly after club feet and spina bifida, 50% lip and palate involvement, 25% palate alone, and 25% lip alone

S+S

- Cleft of lip, cleft on palate
- Cleft palate associated with feeding difficulty: choking from milk entering the nose

Complications

- Secretory otitis media, speech problems, Eustachian tube dysfunction, hearing loss

Rx

- Multidisciplinary team management: plastics, ENT surgeon, pediatrician.
- Breastfeeding often successful in affected infants.
- Bottle-fed babies may require special teats and feeding devices.
- Surgical repair of the lip may be performed during first few week of life.
- Surgical repair of palate at several months of age.
- Speech therapy, parent support groups.

Chapter 3

Pulmonology

3.1   Wheezing in Toddlers

General Ref

- *Lancet* 2002;360:1393
- *Pediatrics* 2002;110:e77

Cause

- Viral-induced wheezing, gastroesophageal reflux (causes reflex bronchospasm), foreign body aspiration, vascular rings, laryngeal web, CF, masses, laryngotracheomalacia, chronic lung disease of prematurity (formerly bronchopulmonary dysplasia), habit cough, tuberculosis, lymph node compressing airways

Pathophys

- Depends on the cause

S+S

- Three wheezing phenotypes are identified in children:
  - Transient early wheezing: risk is increased in preterm babies and with maternal smoking. Very common in infancy. Majority are transient early virus associated wheezing (wheezy bronchitis). Not associated with a family hx of asthma or allergies. Due to small airways obstructing more easily during viral-induced inflammation: resolves by 5 yr of age due to increase in airway caliber.

- Nonatopic wheezing: these children have normal lung function early in life but increased wheezing during the first 10 yr of life following a lower respiratory tract infection (e.g., bronchiolitis). Less severe persistent wheezing in this phenotype and sx improve in adolescence.
- IgE-mediated wheezing/atopic asthma: lung function normal at birth but recurrent wheeze develops with allergic sensitization. Atopic wheezers have persistence of sx and decreased lung function later in childhood. There is usually a family hx of atopy.

3.2 Asthma

General Ref

- *National Asthma Education and Prevention Program Expert Panel Report 3: Guidelines*
- www.nhlbi.nih.gov/guidelines/asthma/asthgdln.htm
- *Eur Respir J* 2007;29:56–62

Cause

- Younger than 5 yr: viral illness most common trigger, exercise, inhalant allergens, emotion

Epidem

- Prevalence equal in African American and white children but more severe disease in African Americans
- Mortality highest in African American followed by Latinos then whites; unclear whether ethnic or socioeconomic differences

Pathophys

- Inflammation causes airway hyperresponsiveness, hyperreactivity, and airway obstruction.

S+S

- Recurrent episodes of coughing and/or wheezing, shortness of breath (SOB), and chest tightness; children may cough without wheezing. Cough dry, worse at night, increases with activity.
- Rules of two:
  - Do you use a quick relief inhaler more than twice weekly?
  - Do you wake up with asthma more than twice monthly?
  - Do you refill your short-acting β-agonist more than twice yearly?
- If yes to any of the preceding questions, patient has persistent asthma or poorly controlled asthma.

Course

With appropriate therapy and good adherence to treatment regimen course, prognosis usually excellent.

Lab

- Clinical dx, spirometry, pulmonary function tests

Rx

- Avoid Vicks VapoRub: irritant.
- Stepwise approach for managing asthma long term in children 0–4 yr and 5–11 yr:
  - Avoid triggers.
  - Asthma written action plan (*Cochrane Database Syst Rev* 2006: children using asthma action plan, lower risk of exacerbations requiring acute care visit).
  - Teach pts self-evaluation (*Cochrane* studies show symptom-based plan as accurate as peak flow–based plan).
  - Make sure patient knows how to use inhalers correctly.
  - Make sure timing is correct: montelukast qhs (at bedtime), steroids every morning.
  - Step up and step down appropriately.
  - Patient-initiated oral corticosteroids in select pts.

Table 3.1 Classification of Asthma

Assessing severity and initiating therapy in children who are not currently taking long-term control medication.

Components of Severity			Classification of Asthma Severity (0–4 years of age)			
			Intermittent	Persistent		
				Mild	Moderate	Severe
Impairment		Symptoms	≤ 2 days/week	> 2 days/week but not daily	Daily	Throughout the day
		Nighttime awakenings	0	1–2x/month	3–4x/month	> 1x/week
		Short-acting beta2-agonist use for symptom control (not prevention of EIB)	≤ 2 days/week	> 2 days/week but not daily	Daily	Several times per day
		Interference with normal activity	None	Minor limitation	Some limitation	Extremely limited
Risk		Exacerbations requiring oral systemic corticosteroids	0–1/year	≥ 2 exacerbations in 6 months requiring oral systemic corticosteroids, or ≥ 4 wheezing episodes/1 year lasting > 1 day AND risk factors for persistent asthma		
				Consider severity and interval since last exacerbation. Frequency and severity may fluctuate over time. Exacerbations of any severity may occur in pts in any severity category.		
Recommended Step for Initiating Treatment			Step 1	Step 2	Step 3 and consider short course of oral systemic corticosteroids	
			In 2–6 weeks, depending on severity, evaluate level of asthma control that is achieved. If no clear benefit is observed in 4–6 weeks, consider adjusting therapy or alternative diagnosis.			

Abbreviation: EIB, exercise-induced bronchospasm.

Reprinted with permission from *Expert Panel Report 3 (EPR3): Guidelines for the Diagnosis and Management of Asthma, 2007*. National Heart, Lung, and Blood Institute as part of the National Institutes of Health and the US Department of Health and Human Services.

Table 3.2 Classifying Asthma Severity

Assessing severity and initiating therapy in children who are not currently taking long-term control medication.

Components of Severity		Classification of Asthma Severity (5–11 years of age)			
		Intermittent	Persistent		
			Mild	Moderate	Severe
Impairment	Symptoms	≤ 2 days/week	> 2 days/week but not daily	Daily	Throughout the day
	Nighttime awakenings	≤ 2x/month	3–4x/month	> 1x/week but not nightly	Often 7x/week
	Short-acting beta₂-agonist use for symptom control (not prevention of EIB)	≤ 2 days/week	> 2 days/week but not daily	Daily	Several times per day
	Interference with normal activity	None	Minor limitation	Some limitation	Extremely limited
	Lung function	• Normal FEV1 between exacerbations • FEV_1 > 80% predicted • FEV_1/FVC > 85%	• FEV_1 => 80% predicted • FEV_1/FVC > 80%	• FEV_1 = 60–80% predicted • FEV_1/FVC = 75–80%	• FEV_1 < 60% predicted • FEV_1/FVC < 75%
Risk	Exacerbations requiring oral systemic corticosteroids	0–1/year (see note)	≥ 2/year (see note)		
		Consider severity and interval since last exacerbation. Frequency and severity may fluctuate over time for pts in any severity category. Relative annual risk of exacerbations may be related to FEV_1			
Recommended Step for Initiating Treatment		Step 1	Step 2	Step 3, medium-dose ICS option	Step 3, medium-dose ICS option or step 4
				Step 3, medium-dose ICS option and consider short course of oral systemic corticosteroids	
		In 2–6 weeks, evaluate level of asthma control that is achieved, and adjust therapy accordingly			

Abbreviations: EIB, exercise-induced bronchospasm; FEV1, forced expiratory volume in 1 second; FVC, forced vital capacity; ICS, inhaled corticosteroids.
Note: At present, there are inadequate data to correspond frequencies of exacerbations with different levels of asthma severity. In general, more frequent and intense exacerbations (e.g., requiring urgent, unscheduled care, hospitalization, or ICU admission) indicate greater underlying disease severity. For treatment purposes, pts who had ≥ 2 exacerbations requiring oral systemic corticosteroids in the past year may be considered the same as pts who have persistent asthma, even in the absence of impairment levels consistent with persistent asthma.

Reprinted with permission from *Expert Panel Report 3 (EPR3): Guidelines for the Diagnosis and Management of Asthma, 2007*. National Heart, Lung, and Blood Institute as part of the National Institutes of Health and the US Department of Health and Human Services.

PULMONOLOGY

Table 3.3 Assessing Asthma Control and Adjusting Therapy in Children 0–4 Years of Age

Components of Control		Classification of Asthma Control (0–4 years)		
		Well Controlled	Not Well Controlled	Very Poorly Controlled
Impairment	Symptoms	≤ 2 days/week	> 2 days/week	Throughout the day
	Nighttime awakenings	1x/month	> 1x/month	> 1x/week
	Interference with normal activity	None	Some limitation	Extremely limited
	Short-acting beta$_2$-agonist use for symptom control (not prevention of EIB)	≤ 2 days/week	> 2 days/week	Several times per day
Risk	Exacerbations requiring oral systemic corticosteroids	0–1/year	2–3/year	> 3/year
	Treatment-related adverse effects	Medication side effects can vary in intensity from none to very troublesome and worrisome. The level of intensity does not correlate to specific levels of control but should be considered in the overall assessment of risk.		
Recommended Action for Treatment		• Maintain current treatment • Regular follow up every 1–6 months • Consider step down if well controlled for at least 3 months	• Step up (1 step) and • Reevaluate in 2–6 weeks • If no clear benefit in 4–6 weeks, consider alternative diagnoses or adjusting therapy • For side effects, consider alternative treatment options	• Consider short course of oral systemic corticosteroids • Step up (1–2 steps), and • Reevaluate in 2 weeks • If no clear benefit in 4–6 weeks, consider alternative diagnoses or adjusting therapy • For side effects, consider alternative treatment options

Abbreviation: EIB, exercise-induced bronchospasm.

Reprinted with permission from *Expert Panel Report 3 (EPR3): Guidelines for the Diagnosis and Management of Asthma, 2007.* National Heart, Lung, and Blood Institute as part of the National Institutes of Health and the US Department of Health and Human Services.

Table 3.4 Stepwise Approach for Managing Asthma in Children 0–4 Years of Age

Intermittent Asthma	Persistent Asthma: Daily Medication
	Consult with asthma specialist if step 3 care or higher is required. Consider consultation at step 2.

Step 6
Preferred:
High-dose ICS + either LABA
or
Montelukast
Oral systemic Corticosteroids

Step 5
Preferred:
High-dose ICS + either LABA or Montelukast

Step 4
Preferred:
Medium-dose ICS + either LABA or Montelukast

Step 3
Preferred:
Medium-dose ICS

Step 2
Preferred:
Low-dose ICS
Alternative:
Cromoly nor Montelukast

Step 1
Preferred:
SABA PRN

Step up if needed
(first, check adherence, inhaler technique, and environmental control)

Assess control

Step down if possible
(and asthma is well controlled at least 3 months)

Patient Education and Environmental Control at Each Step

Quick-relief medication for all pts.
SABA as needed for symptoms. Intensity of treatment depends on severity of symptoms.
With viral respiratory infection: SABA q 4-6 hours up to 24 hours (longer with physician consult). Consider short course of oral systemic corticosteroids if exacerbation is severe or patient has history of previous severe exacerbations.
Caution: Frequent use of SABA may indicate the need to step up treatment. See text for recommendations on initiating daily long-term-control therapy.

Abbreviation: Alphabetical order is used when more than one treatment option is listed within either preferred or alternative therapy. ICS, inhaled corticosteroid; LABA, inhaled long-acting beta₂-agonist; SABA, inhaled short-acting beta₂-agonist.

Reprinted with permission from *Expert Panel Report 3 (EPR3): Guidelines for the Diagnosis and Management of Asthma, 2007.* National Heart, Lung, and Blood Institute as part of the National Institutes of Health and the US Department of Health and Human Services.

PULMONOLOGY

Table 3.5   Assessing Asthma Control and Adjusting Therapy in Children 5–11 Years of Age

Components of Control		Classification of Asthma Control (5–11 years of age)		
		Well Controlled	**Not Well Controlled**	**Very Poorly Controlled**
Impairment	Symptoms	≤ 2 days/week but not more than once on each day	> 2 days/week or multiple times on ≤ 2 days/week	Throughout the day
	Nighttime awakenings	≤ 1x/month	≥ 2x/month	≥ 2x/week
	Interference with normal activity	None	Some limitation	Extremely limited
	Short-acting beta₂-agonist use for symptom control (not prevention of EIB)	≤ 2 days/week	> 2 days/week	Several times per day
	Lung function • FEV or peak flow • FEV₁/FEV	• > 80% predicted/personal best • > 80%	• 60–80% predicted/personal best • 75–80%	• < 60% predicted/personal best • < 75%
Risk	Exacerbations requiring oral systemic corticosteroids	0–1/year	Consider severity and interval since last exacerbation.	≥ 2/year (see note)
	Reduction in lung growth	Evaluation requires long-term follow-up.		
	Treatment-related adverse effects	Medication side effects can vary in intensity from none to very troublesome and worrisome. The level of intensity does not correlate to specific levels of control but should be considered in the overall assessment of risk.		
Recommended Action for Treatment		• Maintain current step • Regular follow up every 1–6 months • Consider step down if well controlled for at least 3 months	• Step up at least 1 step, and • Reevaluate in 2–6 weeks • For side effects, consider alternative treatment options	• Consider short course of oral systemic corticosteroids • Step up 1–2 steps and • Reevaluate in 2 weeks • For side effects, consider alternative treatment options

Abbreviations: EIB, exercise-induced bronchospasm; FEV1, forced expiratory volume in 1 second; FVC, forced vital capacity.
Note: At present, there are inadequate data to correspond frequencies of exacerbations with different levels of asthma severity. In general, more frequent and intense exacerbations (e.g., requiring urgent, unscheduled care, hospitalization, or ICU admission) indicate greater underlying disease severity. For treatment purposes, pts who had ≥ 2 exacerbations requiring oral systemic corticosteroids in the past year may be considered the same as pts who have persistent asthma, evenin the absence of impairment levels consistent with persistent asthma.

Reprinted with permission from *Expert Panel Report 3 (EPR3): Guidelines for the Diagnosis and Management of Asthma, 2007.* National Heart, Lung, and Blood Institute as part of the National Institutes of Health and the US Department of Health and Human Services.

Table 3.6 Stepwise Approach for Managing Asthma in Children 5–11 Years of Age

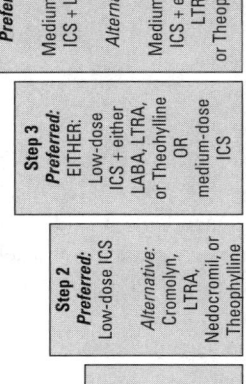

Intermittent Asthma	Persistent Asthma: Daily Medication Consult with asthma specialist if step 4 care or higher is required. Consider consultation at step 3.					Step up if needed (first, check adherence, inhaler technique, environmental control, and comorbid conditions) *Assess control* Step down if possible (and asthma is well controlled at least 3 months)
Step 1 ***Preferred:*** SABA PRN	**Step 2** ***Preferred:*** Low-dose ICS *Alternative:* Cromolyn, LTRA, Nedocromil, or Theophylline	**Step 3** ***Preferred:*** EITHER: Low-dose ICS + either LABA, LTRA, or Theophylline OR medium-dose ICS	**Step 4** ***Preferred:*** Medium-dose ICS + LABA *Alternative:* Medium-dose ICS + either LTRA or Theophylline	**Step 5** ***Preferred:*** High-dose ICS + LABA *Alternative:* High-dose ICS + either LTRA or Theophylline	**Step 6** ***Preferred:*** High-dose ICS + LABA + oral systemic corticosteroid *Alternative:* High-dose ICS + either LTRA or Theophylline + oral systemic corticosteroid	

Each step: Patient education, environmental control, and management of comorbidities.*

Steps 2–4: Consider subcutaneous allergen immunotherapy for pts who have allergic asthma.

Quick-relief medication for all pts.

SABA as needed for symptoms. Intensity of treatment depends on severity of symptoms: up to 3 treatments at 20-minute intervals as needed. Short course of oral systemic corticosteroids may be needed.

Caution: Increasing use of SABA or use > 2 days a week for symptom relief (not prevention of EIB) generally indicates inadequate control and the need to step up treatment.

Abbreviations: Alphabetical order is used when more than one treatment option is listed within either preferred or alternative therapy; ICS, inhaled corticosteroid; LABA, inhaled long-acting beta₂-agonist; LTRA, leukotriene receptor antagonist; SABA, inhaled short-acting beta₂-agonist.

*Immunotherapy for steps 2–4 is based on Evidence B for house-dust mites, animal danders, and pollens; evidence is weak or lacking for molds and cockroaches. Evidence is strongest for immunotherapy with single allergens. The role of allergy in asthma is greater in children than in adults. Clinicians who administer immunotherapy should be prepared and equipped to identify and treat anaphylaxis that may occur.

Reprinted with permission from *Expert Panel Report 3 (EPR3): Guidelines for the Diagnosis and Management of Asthma, 2007.* National Heart, Lung, and Blood Institute as part of the National Institutes of Health and the US Department of Health and Human Services.

PULMONOLOGY

3.3   Cystic Fibrosis

General Ref

- *Lancet* 2003;361:681–689
- *JAMA* 2009;302:1076–1078

Cause

- Autosomal recessive.
- Defective gene on chromosome 7 that codes for CFTR.
- More than 1500 gene mutations have been discovered in CF; deltaF508 found in 75% of cases.

Epidem

- Most common fatal inherited disorder in whites
- Whites carrier rate 1 in 25, with 1 in 3500 affected births; less common in other ethnic groups
- More than 30,000 affected individuals in the United States with more than 1000 newly diagnosed cases each year

Pathophys

- Deficiency of CFTR causes failure of chloride secretion and excessive sodium reabsorption.
- CFTR is a cAMP-dependent chloride channel blocker.
- Abnormal ion transport across the epithelial cells of exocrine glands of the respiratory tract and pancreas results in increased viscosity of secretions.
- Excessive NaCl concentration from abnormal function of sweat glands.

S+S

- Pulmonary: recurrent respiratory tract infections, pneumonia, clubbing, chronic obstructive pulmonary disease. Less com-

mon: nasal polyps, allergic bronchopulmonary aspergillosis, pseudomonas bronchitis
- Gastrointestinal: meconium ileus: 10%, pathognomonic, FTT, steatorrhea and malabsorption in > 90%, and deficiency of fat-soluble vitamins D, A, K, and E.
- Obstructive jaundice, rectal prolapse: may be presenting complaint; hypoproteinemia. Less common: pancreatitis, bronchiectasis, and prolonged cholestasis.
- Endocrine: insidious onset of DM usually requiring insulin.
- Genitourinary tract: congenital bilateral absence of the vas deferens resulting in male infertility.
- Sweat gland obstruction: inability to lose heat, heat exhaustion.

Course

- Median life expectancy: 40 yr

Lab

- Immunoreactive trypsinogen (IRT)
- Sweat test: Na and Cl concentrations > 60 mEq/L diagnostic
- Genotyping for CFTR

Rx

- Goals: multidisciplinary team working to prevent lung disease, promote nutrition, treat complications
- Daily chest physiotherapy
- Continuous oral antibiotics with IV as needed
- Nebulized antibiotics in chronic infections
- Dietary counseling and pancreatic enzyme supplements
- Studies into gene therapy ongoing and provide possible future treatment modality; *Hum Gene Ther* 2004;15:1255–1269

3.4   Pneumonia

General Ref

- *N Engl J Med* 2002;346:429

Cause

- Varies with age:
  - Neonates: group B streptococcus, *Escherichia coli*, entero-cocci, *Listeria monocytogenes*
  - Infants and young children: Respiratory syncytial virus (RSV), pneumococcus, *Haemophilus influenzae*, *Chlamydia trachomatis*, *Bordetella pertussis*, *Staphylococcus aureus* (rare but serious)
  - Children > 5 yr: pneumococcus, mycoplasma, *Chlamydia*, *Legionella*

Epidem

- Incidence highest in infancy

S+S

- Fever, chills, hypothermia in neonates, shortness of breath, cough (paroxysmal with posttussive vomiting in pertussis), lethargy, poor feeding; apnea may be seen infants with pertussis.

Course

- Virtually all children make a full recovery.

Complications

- Empyema, pleural effusion, pneumothorax, sepsis, lung abscess

Lab

- Nasopharyngeal aspirate
- CBC and acute phase reactants generally unhelpful in distinguishing between viral and bacterial pneumonia

- Blood cultures if < 3 months of age or immunocompromised
- PPD if TB is suspected

Imaging

- Chest Xray (follow-up chest Xray at 4–6 wk indicated if collapse or empyema)
- Chest ultrasound/chest CT distinguishes parapneumonic effusion from empyema

Rx

- Outpatient management: Most cases are mild and can be managed at home. Outpatient antibiotic choices:
    - Younger than 5 yr atypical pneumonia uncommon:
        - Amoxicillin: 45–90 mg/kg per day divided twice or three times daily
        - Cefdinir: 14 mg/kg/day divided daily or twice daily
        - Cefuroxime: 30 mg/kg per day divided twice daily
        - Cefpodoxime: 10 mg/kg per day divided twice daily
    - Older than 5 yr: atypical pathogens much more common:
        - Erythromycin 30–50 mg/kg per day divided three or four times daily.
        - May also use azithromycin or other macrolides.
        - Tetracyclines may be used in children > 9 yr.
        - Fluoroquinolones may be used in adolescents > 16 yr.
- Inpatient management:
    - Consider if oxygen saturations less than 93% or signs of respiratory distress
    - Oxygen to keep saturations more than 95%
    - Children > 2 months:
        - Ampicillin 200 mg/kg per day divided twice or three times daily plus gentamicin 6 mg/kg per day divided three times daily

- Children 2 months to 5 yr:
  - Ceftriaxone 50–75 mg/kg per day divided twice daily or daily.
  - Cefuroxime 75–150 mg/kg per day divided 3 times a day.
  - Cefotaxime 100–200 mg/kg per day divided 3 or 4 times a day.
  - Add vancomycin 60 mg/kg per day divided 4 times a day if seriously ill.
  - Oxacillin, cefazolin, nafcillin, or clindamycin can all be considered if staphylococcal coverage indicates.
- Children ≥ 5 years or older:
  - Erythromycin or azithromycin should be included for atypical coverage.

3.5 Bronchiolitis

General Ref

- AAP guidelines
- *Pediatrics* 2007;119:e70–76
- *Arch Pediatr Adolesc Med* 2004;158:119–126

Cause

- Ref: *Acad Emerg Med* 2008;15:111–118
- RSV 70%
- Human metapneumovirus 10–20%
- Parainfluenza, adenovirus, rhinovirus all cause about 2%

Epidem

- Fall through winter, most children infected with RSV by 2 yr of age; 3% requiring hospitalization; incubation period 2–8 d.

Pathophys

- Viral infection of lower respiratory tract characterized by acute inflammation, edema, and necrosis of epithelial cells lining small airways, with increased mucus production and bronchospasm

S+S

- Most children get upper respiratory prodrome sx only, with rhinorrhea, coryza, and cough.
- Some go on to wheezing.
- A small percentage of pts develop tachypnea and signs of respiratory distress.

Course

- Mortality close to zero

Lab

- Routine labs and Xray not usually needed. Diagnosis is clinical.
- Nasopharyngeal swabs.
- RSV serology.
- Pulse oximetry; ABG analysis.

Imaging

- Chest Xray: hyperinflation, patchy atelectasis, diffuse interstitial infiltrates

Rx

- Supportive measures: hydration, supplemental oxygen, suction of upper airways.
- Bronchodilators should not be used routinely; trial an option but only continue if objective clinical improvement (improved respiratory rate and oxygen saturations); 57% improve

(43% improve with placebo); does not affect the outcome or prevent admission.
- No difference between racemic epinephrine and albuterol; no place in the outpatient setting.
- No role for steroids (*N Engl J Med* July 2007).
- Studies suggest hypertonic saline nebulizer treatments may improve sx (*J Pediatr* September 2007).
- Aerosolized ribavirin speeds recovery in ventilated children with RSV.
- Prevention: high-risk children (e.g., chronic lung disease, prematurity < 32 weeks gestational age, congenital heart disease). Palivizumab (Synagis), a monoclonal antibody, can be given in RSV season (*Med Lett* 2001;43:13); maximum number of doses: 5.

3.6 Allergic Rhinitis

General Ref
- *Immunol Allergy Clin North Am* 2005;25:301–312
- *Am J Respir Crit Care Med* 2007;176:659–666

Cause
- House-dust mites, molds, animal dander, tree pollens, grass

Epidem
- Perennial allergic rhinitis occurs at any age; seasonal allergic rhinitis rare in children < 3 yr.
- Begins in childhood and peaks in adolescence; 80% of cases occur in adolescents < 20 yr.
- Most common allergic condition in the United States.
- 75% children with asthma also have allergic rhinitis; increased incidence if family hx of atopy.

S+S

- Itching, sneezing, clear rhinorrhea, conjunctival irritation, nasal congestion more at night, allergic shiners (dark circles under the eyes), transverse nasal crease, conjunctival edema, tearing
- Associated with sinusitis, otitis media, eczema, and asthma

Course

- Limited data, but studies suggest that although some children will have improvement of symptoms with age, many will have persistent and sometimes worsening symptoms.

Lab

- Epicutaneous skin tests detect allergen-specific IgE.
- Serum immunoassay alternative test for allergen-specific IgE.
- Eosinophil count in nasal smear.
- CBC and differential may show eosinophilia.

Rx

- Identify and eliminate known allergens.
- Antihistamines for itching and sneezing; second-generation drugs have fewer CNS side effects: loratadine (Claritin), cetirizine (Zyrtec), fexofenadine (Allegra).
- Intranasal steroids: Must be used regularly because may take up to 2 wk to be fully effective:
  - Beclomethasone (Beconase), budesonide (Rhinocort), and flunisolide (AeroBid) may be used in children $\geq$ 6 yr.
  - Fluticasone propionate (Flonase 0.05%) may be used in children $\geq$ 4 yr.
  - Mometasone furoate monohydrate (Nasonex) may be used in children $\geq$ 2 yr.

- Immunotherapy (desensitization) considered if no response to pharmacologic treatment. Sublingual immunotherapy currently used widely in Europe; not yet approved by FDA in the United States (*Allergy Asthma Proc* 2007;28:1).

3.7 Croup

General Ref

- *Cochrane Database Syst Rev* 2004;1:CD001955

Cause

- Parainfluenza virus type 1 most common; other organisms include RSV, influenza, adenovirus, enterovirus, metapneumovirus, mycoplasma pneumoniae.

Epidem

- M:F ratio: 3:2
- Younger children in first 3 yr of life with a peak in 2nd year
- Occurs in the fall and early winter
- Incubation period: 2–6 d

Pathophys

- Spread via droplet nuclei; airway narrowing occurs as a result of increased mucus production, with edema of the subglottic space and vocal cords causing the predominant signs of upper airway obstruction.

S+S

- Prodrome of upper respiratory sx, sore throat, fever, then barking cough and stridor. Mild disease: barking cough with no stridor progressing to stridor with agitation, stridor at rest, and most severe, signs of respiratory distress with retractions and cyanosis.

Course

- Uneventful course; most cases do not require hospitalization.

Complications

- Dehydration, upper airway obstruction, respiratory failure (rare)

Lab

- Usually clinical dx
- CBC not particularly helpful in dx (in severe cases blood draws may agitate child so avoid)

Imaging

- Anteroposterior neck views: "steeple sign"
- Lateral neck Xrays show subglottic narrowing with a normal epiglottis (not needed in a child with classic presentation)

Rx

- Most managed supportively at home:
  - Mild: oral hydration and minimal handling
  - Moderate to severe:
    - Dexamethasone 0.6 mg/kg im or po for one dose. Improves sx, decreases hospital stay, decreases frequency of intubation (some studies suggest single dose of 0.15 mg/kg as effective as 0.6 mg; no evidence to support multiple doses).
    - Racemic epinephrine causes immediate reduction in swelling of laryngeal airway in a child in acute distress.
  - Impending respiratory failure: prompt intubation; do not wait for Xrays to confirm dx.

3.8 Tuberculosis

General Ref

- *Pediatr Infect Dis J* 2006;25:941
- *Lancet* 2006;367:938–940

Cause

- *Mycobacterium tuberculosis* complex (M. *tuberculosis*, M. *bovis*, and M. *africanum*), a closely related group of acid-fast bacilli

Epidem

- Higher incidence with low socioeconomic conditions; two-thirds of reported cases in United States occur in nonwhite racial group.
- Incubation period: 2–12 wk (from infection to development of positive tuberculin skin test).

Pathophys

- Defects in interferon gamma and IL-12 pathways predispose to infection (JAMA 2001;286:1740).
- Infection is usually via respiratory route.
- Bacteria are ingested by pulmonary macrophages.
- A cellular immune response is mounted.
- Healing of the pulmonary foci occurs that calcifies into the Ghon focus.
- Surviving bacilli remain dormant and may reactivate in later life causing smear-positive tuberculous disease.

S+S

- Fever, malaise, anorexia, weight loss, cough, night sweats
- Hypersensitivity reactions: erythema nodosum, phlyctenular conjunctivitis
- Dissemination more common in children > 4 yr: miliary TB, TB meningitis, TB of bones and joints, TB pericarditis

Lab

- Zeihl-Neelsen staining of the following:
  - Early morning gastric washings on 3 consecutive mornings
  - Bronchoalveolar lavage fluid
  - CSF
  - Urine
- Positive PPD.
- PCRs have poor sensitivity and specificity
- Interferon gamma release assay (IGRAs)—in vitro blood tests of cell mediated immune response greater specificity than skin tests and can be used on pts that have had BCG—still limited data on use in children (*Thorax* 2006;61(7):616–620; *Ann Intern Med* 2008;149(3):177–184).

Pathophys

- Lymph node bx will show caseating granulomata.

Imaging

- Chest Xray: typically hilar lymphadenopathy and parenchymal changes

Rx

- Triple or quadruple therapy with rifampicin, isoniazid, pyrazinamide, and ethambutol for 2 months followed by a 2-drug regimen of rifampicin and isoniazid for a further 4 months
- Weekly pyridoxine is added after puberty to help prevent the peripheral neuropathy associated with isoniazid. This complication is not seen in young children.
- Asymptomatic PPD-positive children are treated with 3 months of rifampicin and isoniazid.

Chapter 4

Infectious Diseases

4.1 Fever Without a Source

General Ref

- *Arch Dis Child* 2009;94:144
- *Ann Emerg Med* 1993;22:1198–1210
- *Pediatrics* 1999;103:627–631

Def

- Fever without a source (FWS): fever of ≤ 1 wk duration, unexplained by full H+P; need full evaluation and often empirical antibiotics.
- Fever of unknown origin (FUO): children with fever of at least 8 days' duration in whom no dx is apparent after initial inpatient or outpatient evaluation. Assessment is not emergent, and antibiotics are usually not indicated.

Cause

- Infections the most common cause. A cause is often never found.

Epidem

- Rates of occult bacteremia have decreased significantly due to successful immunization programs.

S+S

- May be well appearing with just a fever; ill-appearing infants may be lethargic, irritable, have a high-pitched cry. Studies consistently show that if these children have no respiratory sx. Chest Xray is usually normal, so usually only helpful if associated clinical sign, such as tachypnea, grunting, rales, retractions, or nasal flaring.

Lab

- CBC and differential, peripheral blood smear, blood culture
- LP as part of workup if infant < 28 d or if ill appearing in older infants
- ESR and CRP
- UA and culture
- Electrolytes, BUN and creatinine, LFTs
- HIV serology
- Chest Xray, PPD
- Further labs if indicated by H+P

Rx

- The following children presenting with FWS should be hospitalized and managed with parenteral antibiotics:
  - All infants < 28 d regardless of clinical picture with rectal temperature ≥ 38°C:
    - Treat with parenteral ampicillin and gentamicin or ampicillin and cefotaxime.
    - Add acyclovir 60 mg/kg per day divided 3 times a day if seizures or mucocutaneous vesicles.
  - All toxic-appearing infants 29–90 d of age:
    - Treat with IV ceftriaxone or cefotaxime.
    - If the infant has CSF pleocytosis or is sick looking, treat with ampicillin, ceftriaxone (or cefotaxime), and vancomycin.

- Children 3–36 months of age with fever > 39°C, WBC > 15,000/μL:
  - Treat with parenteral antibiotics pending blood culture and urine culture results, ceftriaxone 50 mg/kg IV daily. (If allergy to cephalosporins: clindamycin 10 mg/kg IV followed by po 8 hr later.)
  - Any child in whom concerned caregiver may not recognize signs of deteriorating sx.
  - Children may be discharged if clinically well and blood cultures have been negative for 24–48 hr (*Pediatrics* 2000;106:251–255).
- The following children may be managed in the outpatient setting (*Pediatrics* 1999;103:627–631):
  - Nontoxic febrile infants 28–90 d, with low-risk clinical and lab picture and close follow-up assured.
  - Children > 3 months with FWS < 39°C do not need labs or antibiotics.
  - In a fully immunized child the risk of occult bacteremia is < 1%, no labs or antibiotics indicated, UTI most likely source and UA and urine cultures indicated (*Arch Dis Child* 2009;94:144).
  - Urine culture should be obtained from all boys ≤ 6 months and girls ≤ 2 yr.
  - Caregiver must be advised to seek medical attention if fever persists for > 48 hr in above setting or clinical picture deteriorates.

4.2   Cat Scratch Disease

General Ref

- *Pediatr Infect Dis J* 2000;19:1185
- *N Engl J Med* 1997;337:1876

Cause

- *Bartonella henselae*, a gram-negative bacillus.
- Infection follows cat scratch or contact with a cat or kitten.
- The cat or kitten is usually healthy.

Epidem

- Worldwide distribution
- 20,000 cases per year in United States
- More common in fall and winter

S+S

- Primary lesion (papule or pustule) at wound site following a 3- to 10-d incubation period, followed by regional lymphadenopathy (40% suppurative), headache, fever, malaise

Course

- Benign, self-limiting. Prognosis good if no complications.

Complications

- Encephalitis, parotid swelling, erythema nodosum, pneumonia, granuloma of liver and spleen, endocarditis (*Ann Intern Med* 1996;125:646).
- Immunocompromised individuals may develop bacillary angiomatosis (*N Engl J Med* 1997;337:1876, 1888, 1916), vascular tumors of skin and subcutaneous tissue.

Lab

- Increased WCC with left shift, mildly elevated eosinophils
- Elevated ESR

CNS Involvement

- CSF: slight increase in protein with mononuclear cells

Histopathology

- Pyogenic granulomas; organisms demonstrated by Warthin-Starry and silver stains
- Serology: ELISA: titers > 1:64, indirect fluorescent antibody testing, PCR

Rx

- Reassurance; usually resolves without treatment in mild disease.
- 5-d azithromycin has been shown to speed resolution of lymphadenopathy.
- Individuals with disseminated disease often require treatment.
- Immunocompromised individuals often need long-term therapy to prevent recurrence: doxycycline, macrolides, ciprofloxacin, or gentamicin may be used.

4.3   Acute Otitis Media

General Ref

- *Pediatrics* 2004;113:1451–1465
- *Lancet* 2004;363:465–473

Cause

- *Haemophilus* influenza, pneumococcus, *Moraxella catarrhalis*, *Streptococcus*, viral

Epidem

- More common in fall and winter; peak incidence 6–12 months

Pathophys

- Eustachian tube dysfunction: shorter and more horizontal in younger children and function poorly.

INFECTIOUS DISEASES

S+S

- Sx: fever, feeling of fullness, pain that may improve with spontaneous drainage
- Si: bulging tympanic membrane, loss of light reflex, poor air movement and pain with pneumatic otoscopy, decreased hearing

Course

- May resolve without antibiotics; improves within 48 hr of antibiotics

Protective Factors

- Breastfeeding protects against otitis media in 1st yr of life.
- Delaying day care or choosing day care with $\leq$ 5 children, thus decreasing exposure to respiratory pathogens.
- Avoiding secondhand smoke exposure.
- Influenza vaccine.

Complications

- Serious complications such as mastoiditis and meningitis are now uncommon.

Lab

- Tympanometry

Rx

- Acetaminophen or ibuprofen for pain.
- 80% of cases resolve spontaneously.
- Antibiotics shorten the duration of pain but do not decrease risk of hearing loss.
- High-dose amoxicillin 80–90 mg/kg per day is drug of choice. Treat for 5 d; if prior AOM within past month, treat for 10 d.
- Second-line drugs: cefdinir, cefpodoxime, cefuroxime.
- No evidence of benefit from decongestant or antihistamine.

4.4   Otitis Media with Effusion

General Ref

- *Pediatrics* 2004;113:1412–1429
- *Arch Pediatr Adolesc Med* 2001;155:1137–1142

Cause

- Fluid secretion without culturable organisms

Epidem

- Peak incidence: 1 yr

Pathophys

- Chronic inflammation with the proliferation of mucous-secreting goblet cells. Altered ciliary function, allergies, and gastroesophageal reflux have all been suggested as contributing to OME.

S+S

- Asymptomatic apart from possible decreased hearing. Tympanic membrane is dull and retracted.

Course

- Pt with persistent otitis media > 3 months may have hearing loss.

Complications

- Most common cause of conductive hearing loss in children
- May result in disturbed speech development and learning difficulties

Rx

- Usually resolves spontaneously.
- Consider insertion of grommets and adenoidectomy if hearing loss.

INFECTIOUS DISEASES

4.5 *Streptococcus* Pharyngitis

General Ref

- *Ann Intern Med* 2001;134:506, 509
- *BMJ* 2007;334:939
- *Pediatr Infect Dis J* 2006;25:761–767

Cause

- β-Hemolytic *Streptococcus* group A, rarely C or D, causing intense inflammation of the tonsils

Epidem

- 15% carriers in nasopharynx; spread by droplet nuclei

Pathophys

- Sx: no cough, sore throat, headache, fever
- Si: pharyngeal exudate, tender cervical lymphadenopathy

Course

- 10 d without treatment

Complications

- Poststreptococcal glomerulonephritis, peritonsillar abscess

Lab

- Rapid Strep with culture if negative
- Monospot test

Rx

- Penicillin V or erythromycin (if penicillin allergy) 250 mg po 3 times daily or 4 times daily for 10 d
- Benzathine penicillin 600,000 units im (< 27.2 kg/60 lb) or 1.2 million units im (>27.2 kg/60 lb and adults) for 1 dose

- Avoid amoxicillin: may cause widespread maculopapular rash if the tonsillitis is due to infectious mononucleosis

4.6 Epiglottitis

General Ref

- *Pediatr Clin North Am* 2006;53:215–242
- *Curr Infect Dis Rep* 2008;10:200–204

Cause

- *Haemophilus* influenza type b was the most common pathogen pre-Hib immunizations, but now other bacteria predominate.
- Other organisms: *Streptococcus* group A and C, staphylococcus.

Epidem

- Affects all age groups
- Most common 1–6 yr
- Year-round occurrence
- Male and female predominance equal

Pathophys

- Erythema and edema of the epiglottis, aryepiglottic folds, arytenoids, and hypopharynx with resultant narrowing of the glottic opening

S+S

- Toxic-looking child; sudden onset of fever, dysphagia, drooling, stridor, cyanosis. Child sits, immobile, upright, with an open mouth to optimize the airway.
- Definitive dx via direct visualization of airway: typical cherry red, swollen epiglottis and arytenoids.

Course

- Mortality: 8%

Complications

- Complete airway obstruction, respiratory arrest, hypoxia, and death

Lab

- No blood draws until pt's airway is secured
- CBC: usually elevated; WCC with left shift
- Blood culture

Imaging

- Lateral neck Xrays' "thumbprint sign"; never delay airway intervention for imaging.

Rx

- Medical emergency.
- Manage upright, never supine.
- Oxygen via face mask.
- Anesthetize and intubate under controlled conditions in the operating room.
- Only after airway is secured should blood draws occur.
- IV antibiotics: cefuroxime 150 mg/kg per day divided every 8 hr; alternative IV antibiotics: high-dose penicillin, oxacillin, ampicillin/sulbactam.

4.7 Peritonsillar Abscess

General Ref

- *Am Fam Physician* 2008;77:199–202
- *Pediatr Emerg Care* 2007;23:431–438

Cause

- *Staphylococcus aureus*, *Hemophilias* influenza, group A β-hemolytic streptococci, pneumococcus

Epidem

- Most common in adolescents and adults
- Most common complication of acute tonsillitis
- Most common deep space infection of the head and neck

Pathophys

- Suppurative complication of acute tonsillitis extending into the peritonsillar space

S+S

- High fever, sore throat, dysphagia, drooling, "hot potato" muffled voice

Course

- Complete recovery with appropriate treatment

Complications

- Lateral pharyngeal abscess, risk of airway obstruction, carotid artery erosion, dehydration

Lab

- CBC: elevated WCC with left shift
- Gram stain and culture of aspirate specimen

Rx

- IV hydration
- Analgesia
- IV antibiotics: high-dose IV penicillin first line; second-line antibiotics: clindamycin, cefazolin, oxacillin
- Surgical drainage of abscess

INFECTIOUS DISEASES

4.8 Methicillin-Resistant *Staphylococcus Aureus*

General Ref

- *Pediatr Infect Dis J* 2002;21:431
- *Cochrane Database Syst Rev* 2003;(4):CD003340

Cause

- Staphylococcus: gram positive, nonmotile, aerobic, or facultative anaerobic bacteria. All are catalase positive; *S. aureus* is coagulase positive.
- CA-MRSA (Community-acquired methicillin-resistant *S. aureus* [MRSA])
  - Diagnosed in individuals in whom MRSA is grown in outpatient setting with absent risk factor for nosocomial infection.
  - PCR of CA-MRSA reveals unique genes SCCmec IV and V that code for methicillin resistance.
  - This organism is susceptible to most non-β-lactam antibiotics.
  - Transmission is seen in day-care centers and via contact sports.
  - Has similar presentation to CA-MSSA (methicillin-sensitive *S. aureus*).
  - PVL gene encodes for a leucocidin protein that renders leucocytes less able to deal with staphylococcus infection and so is associated with increased virulence, invasive infections, necrotizing pneumonia, severe infections.
- HA-MRSA (hospital-acquired MRSA):
  - SCCmec types I to III are responsible for methicillin resistance.
  - Multidrug resistance common.

Epidem

- Dramatic increase in cases the past few years
- Carried by 10–36% healthy children

- Most commonly colonizing nares and skin
- Can occur sporadically or in epidemics

Pathophys

- Invasion of tissue with tissue destruction, most commonly skin but also bones (osteomyelitis), pneumonia (can cause severe destructive necrotizing pneumonia) from hematogenous spread
- Toxin-mediated staphylococcus scalded skin syndrome caused by exfoliant toxin, food poisoning, toxic shock syndrome, with mucocutaneous manifestations

S+S

- Clinical presentation depends on the mode of entry.
- Skin invasion (e.g., furuncles, carbuncles, cellulitis).
- Hematogenous spread: osteomyelitis: irritability, fever, nausea, vomiting, local warmth and tenderness. Pneumonia: fever, cough, anorexia, tachypnea, dyspnea.
- Toxin production: food poisoning: staph enterocolitis, sudden onset 1–6 hr after ingestion of contaminated food with diarrhea, crampy abdominal pain, nausea; resolution within 8–24 hr.

Lab

- Gram stain from clinical material; gram-positive cocci in clusters.
- At least 2 blood cultures.
- Food poisoning is a clinical dx; no labs are needed.

Rx

- Mild illness: po antibiotics
- CA-MRSA: linezolid, doxycycline, clindamycin
- HA-MRSA: vancomycin, linezolid, gentamicin plus vancomycin, daptomycin

4.9   Cytomegalovirus Infection

General Ref

- *Pediatrics:* Osborne, p.1388
- *J Pediatr* 2008;53:84

Def

- Complex DNA virus in herpesvirus family; typically harmless in immunocompetent host; problem for neonates, HIV, and transplant recipients

Epidem

- 1–2% of population infected annually, nearly everyone by late adult years.
- 10–20% annual infection rate among uninfected child-care workers.
- Vertical transmission rate in pregnancy is 50% if mother experiences primary infection; 2% vertical transmission rate if infected prior to pregnancy.
- 10% of seropositive mothers have CMV in vaginal secretions; 25–50% excrete CMV in breast milk. Both routes cause symptomless infection in healthy infants but may infect premature infants.
- CMV also present in blood and semen.
- Neonatal disease:
  - 10% symptomatic at birth; one-third of symptomatic CMV infants premature.
  - Asymptomatic infants may have neurologic impairment, typically sensorineural hearing loss (SNHL); serial audiologic screening appropriate for all CMV-infected infants.
  - Disease incidence and severity higher with primary maternal infection.
  - Classic severely affected neonate is "blueberry muffin" baby.

- Si/sx: hepatosplenomegaly, microcephaly, direct jaundice, elevated LFTs, hypotonia, seizures, chorioretinitis, and SNHL (present at birth or progressive later on) all possible.
- 25–30% of congenital CMV infants have enamel defects: yellow, chip easily.
- Dx most easily made by growing virus in urine in infant < 3 wk or positive PCR in blood.
- Ophthalmologic exam may show typical chorioretinitis; CT may show classic calcifications.
- Because clinically overlaps other toxoplasmosis, other infections, rubella, CMV, and herpes simplex syndromes, experts recommend rapid plasma reagin and toxoserology to r/o alternatives.
- No current consensus whether antivirals are of benefit.
- Disease in immunocompetent host:
  - Typically asymptomatic; may present with mononucleosis-like syndrome with atypical lymphs.
  - More rarely, may lead to migrating polyarthritis or pneumonia.
  - Can be prolonged nonspecific febrile illness; self-limited
  - Dx made by serology.
- Immunocompromised host:
  - Si/sx: fever, pneumonia, lymphadenopathy, hepatitis, gi sx, encephalopathy, retinitis all possible.
  - Dx more difficult; requires histologic changes, PCR showing high viral load in body fluid or tissue.
  - R/o *Pneumocystis* and other opportunistic infections.
  - Treatment protocols use ganciclovir along with hyperimmune globulin.

Prevention

- CMV negative blood for seronegative immunocompromised pts. For seronegative mothers, assume all children < 3 yr are

excreting virus; practice good handwashing after contact with
stool, urine, saliva (e.g., diapers, laundry, toys, eating utensils).
- If proven primary infection, hyperimmune globulin can lower
rates of vertical transmission and disease.

4.10   Human Immunodeficiency Virus

General Ref
- *Pediatrics* 2007;120:e1547–e1562
- *Pediatrics* 2009;123:175–187

Cause
- Cytopathic lentivirus and member of the retrovirus family.
HIV 1 and 2 are the etiologic agents. Mother-to-child trans-
mission (MTCT) risk factors:
  - Breastfeeding: 15%
  - Perinatal risk: 5–20% in utero
  - Increased risk with vaginal delivery, especially if rupture of
  membranes is > 8 hr
  - Low CD4 counts and high viral loads in mother
  - Prematurity and chorioamnionitis

Epidem
- HIV 1 much more common in United States than HIV 2.
- Humans are the only reservoirs.

Pathophys
- An acquired defect of cellular immunity associated with infection by HIV
- Lymphocyte count under 200 cells/μL or less than 14% of
total lymphocytes
- Increased susceptibility to opportunistic infections and malignant neoplasms

S + S

- Wasting, opportunistic infection, lymphadenopathy, parotitis, lymphocytic interstitial pneumonitis, *Pneumocystis* pneumonia, recurrent severe thrush, recurrent and chronic diarrhea, acquired microcephaly.
- Clinical manifestations also include emaciation (wasting) and dementia. These elements reflect criteria for AIDS as defined by the CDC in 1993.

Course

- MTCT decreased from 30% to < 1% by the following:
  - Giving antiretroviral therapy (ART) to mother in pregnancy to decrease viral load to < 50,000
  - Delivering baby by lower uterine segment Cesarean section
  - Giving ART to baby first 4–6 wk of life
  - Avoiding breastfeeding
  - Median survival now late teens and adulthood

Lab

- ELISA: repeatedly reactive ELISA in infant < 18 months confirmed by a Western blot is diagnostic (maternal antibodies may be detected up to 15 months of age).
- ELISA performed after 4 wk has > 95% sensitivity and specificity in infancy.
- CD4 counts, CBC, and LFTs taken at dx and every 1–3 months.
- Viral load and baseline CT/MRI of the head for cerebral atrophy repeated annually.

Rx

- Standard immunizations unless symptomatic or very low CD4 counts; then varicella and MMR not given.
- Yearly influenza A and B vaccines.

- Prophylaxis against common opportunistic infections.
- ART: 3 or more antiretroviral drugs.
- Psychosocial support.

4.11 Lyme Disease

General Ref

- *Infect Dis Clin North Am* 2008;22:315–326
- *Pediatrics* 2009;123:959–965
- *Pediatrics* 2009;123:e829–e834

Cause

- Acute and chronic disease complex caused by *Borrelia burgdorferi* inoculated by deer ticks of the *Ixodes* species

Epidem

- Most common tick-borne disease in the United States

Pathophys

- Spirochete disseminated through bloodstream and lymphatics following bite from infected deer tick
- Prolonged tick attachment (24–48 hr) required for transmission of disease

S+S

- Localized infection: bull's-eye rash of erythema chronicum migrans in about 80% of infected pts, flulike sx, headache, muscle soreness, fever and malaise.
- Disseminated infection: migrating pain in muscles, joints, tendons, palpitations and dizziness. Acute neurologic problems occur in 15% of untreated pts. Bell's palsy, meningitis, mild

encephalitis may lead to memory loss, sleep disturbances, or changes in mood or affect.

- Late infection: after several months, untreated or inadequately treated pts may go on to develop severe and chronic sx affecting many organs of the body, including the brain, nerves, eyes, joints, and heart. Lyme disease can progress to later stages even in pts who do not develop a rash.

Course

- Residual arthralgias, fatigue, and memory problems. Course more benign in children.

Complications

- Arthritis, heart block, palpitations, myocarditis, encephalomyelitis, Bell's palsy

Lab

- Serology: B. *burgdorferi* specific increased IgM at 3–4 wk, peaks at 6–8 wk, with increased IgG wk to months later.
- If ELISA is positive, confirm with Western blot.

Rx

- Surveillance: check for ticks and remove to ensure not attached for > 24 hr.
- Localized infection: doxycycline 14–21 d for children > 8 yr; amoxicillin for children < 8 yr.
- Disseminated disease: Extend duration of antibiotics to 21–28 d.
- Recurrent arthritis or carditis may be treated with ceftriaxone for 14–28 d or parenteral penicillin.
- With CNS involvement, treat for 30–60 d.

4.12   Urinary Tract Infection

General Ref

- *Am Fam Physician* 2000;62:1815–1822
- *Cochrane Database Syst Rev* 2004;(4):CD001534
- *Cochrane Database Syst Rev* 2004;(3):CD001532

Cause

- *Escherichia coli* most common organism: 80%
- *Klebsiella, Enterococcus, Proteus mirabilis*
- Following conditions predispose to UTI: posterior urethral valves, bladder diverticulum, voiding dysfunction, vesicoureteric reflux
- Risk factors: constipation, encopresis, bladder instability, infrequent voiding

Epidem

- Most common serious bacterial illness in young children, highest rate in 1st yr of life, more common in uncircumcised boys, more common in white. By 7 yr of age, 8% of girls and 2% of boys have had a UTI.

S+S

- In early childhood, nonspecific sx: fever, lethargy, vomiting, diarrhea, anorexia, irritability. Older children: classic sx of suprapubic discomfort, urgency, frequency, dysuria, hematuria.

Course

- Prompt treatment reduces risk of scarring and its sequelae.

Complications

- Renal scarring, chronic renal failure, HT

Lab

- Ref: *Pediatrics* 1999;104:e54; *Pediatr Infect Dis J* 2002;21:1
- Single organism identified on culture:
  - Suprapubic aspirate > 1000 cfu/mL
  - Catheter specimen > 10,000 cfu/mL
  - Clean catch specimen > 100,000 cfu/mL
  - Urine bags not recommended
- UA:
  - Not helpful if clinical suspicion high (i.e., older children with classic sx)
  - Useful if low likelihood of UTI:
    - Nondilute urine (specific gravity > 1.005)
    - Negative nitrate and leukocyte esterase
    - Negative predictive value > 95%
  - Blood cultures not useful

Imaging

- AAP (American Academy of Pediatrics) recommends imaging:
  - All children 2 months to 2 yr of age with first UTI
  - All boys
  - Girls < 36 months
  - Girls 3–7 yr with fever > 38.5°C (101.3°F)
- Renal US: shows genitourinary tract anatomy and evaluates renal scars; should be done within 6 wk of a UTI, not during the acute phase.
- DMSA: renal cortical scan: differentiates pyelonephritis from cystitis; assesses renal scarring.
- Cystograms: identify and grade vesicoureteric reflux.
- Voiding cystourethrogram: can be used in girls and boys; demonstrates the genitourinary anatomy and identifies any reflux.
- Radionuclide cystogram: can only be used in girls.

Rx

- Trimethoprim/sulfamethoxazole (Bactrim): 6–12 mg/kg and 30–60 mg/kg in 2 doses
- Cefixime (Suprax): 8 mg/kg in 2 doses
- Cefpodoxime (Vantin): 10 mg/kg in 2 doses
- Loracarbef (Lorabid): 15–30 mg/kg in 2 doses

4.13 Cervical Adenitis

General Ref

- *Arch Dis Child* 2003;88:1019
- *Pediatr Infect Dis J* 2009;28:642

Cause

- Bacterial infection: *Streptococcus* and *Staphylococcus* most common. Other causes: MRSA, viral, atypical mycobacteria, tuberculous mycobacteria, *Bartonella henselae*

Epidem

- Most common cause of neck swelling in children > 2 yr, most commonly affecting anterior cervical chain

Pathophys

- Microorganisms penetrate skin of the head and neck and then infiltrate surrounding tissue before being transported to lymph nodes.

S+S

- Tender, enlarged lymph node. May suppurate and form an abscess requiring needle aspiration.
- Cat scratch disease: May present with chronic enlargement, fever, malaise, mildly tender nodes with suppuration within

3–4 wk. There may be a primary papule at scratch site; often no memory of scratch; 90% of cases have hx of contact with a kitten.

- Atypical mycobacterium: caused by mycobacterium avium complex. Mildly tender nodes, unilateral, often matted, overlying skin violaceous.
- Course: Usually self-limiting, cat scratch disease usually resolves in 2 months; may persist for up to 8 months.

Lab

- CBC and differential
- PPD
- Monospot

Imaging

- Chest Xray for hilar adenopathy

Rx

- Early antibiotics may prevent suppuration.
- Needle aspiration if abscess formation.
- Surgical removal if abnormal nodes persist for > 3 months.

4.14   Gastroenteritis

General Ref

- *Arch Dis Child* 1997;77:201
- *Pediatr Rev* 1989;11:6

Cause

- Usually rotavirus; consider *Shigella, Salmonella, Campylobacter* if bloody stools

INFECTIOUS DISEASES

Epidem

- Pathophys (*Arch Dis Child* 1997;77:201): 4 mechanisms:
  - Inflammatory: caused by invasive organisms causing damage to intestinal lining with bloody stools and WBC.
  - Osmotic: Malabsorptive conditions: Unabsorbed substances provide osmotic load, causing water influx.
  - Secretory: Enterotoxins cause increase secretion of fluid and electrolytes via mucosal crypt cells.
  - Cytotoxic: destruction of mucosal small intestinal cells following viral infections.

S+S

- Crampy abdominal pain, following the onset of diarrhea, may be bloody diarrhea; varying signs of dehydration

Complications

- *Campylobacter* associated with Guillain-Barré syndrome.
- Hemolytic uremic syndrome may follow ETEC (enterotoxigenic *E. coli*) 0517.
- Postenteritis enteropathy: lactose intolerance due to loss of intestinal absorptive function.

Lab

- Stool: for culture, ova, parasites, and WCC
- Stool for reducing substances
- *Clostridium difficile* toxin
- Fecal elastase

Rx

- Supportive
- Mild to moderate diarrhea (oral rehydration therapy); IV fluids only if severe or vomiting
- Early refeeding

- No place for use of antidiarrheals in pediatrics
- Antibiotics in dysentery or C. *difficile* infection

4.15 Ehrlichiosis

General Ref

- *Medicine* 2008;87(2):53–60
- *Pediatrics* 2003;112:e252–e253

Cause

- *Ehrlichia sennetsu*, *E. chaffeensis*, *E. phagocytophila*, *E. equi*

Epidem

- Tick-borne infection; *E. chaffeensis* found in Japan and Malaysia; the other types all found in United States. Incubation period 5–10 d following tick bite.

Pathophys

- Intracellular organisms found in polymorphs

S+S

- Fever, chills, headache, nausea, vomiting, cough, arthralgia, myalgia, rash, photophobia, conjunctivitis, pneumonitis, hepatitis, meningitis

Course

- May last several weeks before spontaneous resolution. Mortality < 3%, but may be higher if immunocompromised.

Lab

- CBC: pancytopenia, elevated LFTs
- Immunofluorescent antibody stain available at CDC

Rx

- Doxycycline drug of choice regardless of age (see Rocky Mountain spotted fever); 4 mg/kg per day IV or po divided twice daily for 7–10 d.
- If no improvement within 3 d, consider alternative dx.

4.16   Rocky Mountain Spotted Fever

General Ref

- *Clin Infect Dis* 1995;20:1111–1117

Cause

- *Rickettsia rickettsiae*, an obligate intracellular pathogen
- Reservoirs: dogs and rodents
- Transmitted by lone star tick

Epidem

- Tick-borne disease, endemic in Rocky Mountain rodents, more common on U.S. East Coast; incubation period 2–14 d

Pathophys

- Small vessel vasculitis

S+S

- Fever, headache, photophobia, diarrhea, vomiting, myalgia, splenomegaly, meningismus; rash begins on palms, soles, wrists, and ankles with central spreading.

Course

- Early antibiotic therapy decreases morbidity.

Complications

- 25% fatality in untreated cases; death from vasculitis of heart, lungs, or brain 5–7%

Lab

- CBC: decreased platelet count
- Electrolytes: low sodium, abnormal LFTs
- Serology: Weil Felix

Histopath

- Positive skin biopsy on immunofluorescent stain

Rx

- Tick must be attached for > 6 hr to transmit disease; thus surveillance for ticks and quick removal helps in prevention.
- Doxycycline drug of choice continued for 2–3 d after resolution of fever; minimum of 10 d (expert opinion drug of choice for all age groups: tetracycline; teeth staining is dose dependent, less likely to occur with doxycycline; adverse effects of chloramphenicol more concerning: *Red Book* 2009).
- Alternative drugs: chloramphenicol or fluoroquinolones.

4.17 Pediatric Autoimmune Neuropsychiatric Disorders Associated with *Streptococcus* Infections

General Ref

- *Pediatrics* 2008;121(6):1188–97, 1198–1205

Def

- Pediatric autoimmune neuropsychiatric disorder associated with *Streptococcus* (PANDAS)

- Controversial association between group A strep and acute onset tics or obsessive-compulsive disorder (OCD)

Epidem

- Incidence not known

Sx

- Tic/OCD, pediatric age range (3–16 yr), abrupt onset and episodic course, association with strep infection (culture, antigen test, or antibody), other neurologic sx (hyperactivity, chorea, tics) during exacerbations.
- Sx occur within 1 month of infection.

Clinical Course

- Tics/OCD should clear with treatment and confirms dx.
- Tends to be recurrent.
- Longitudinal studies of PANDAS cases versus chronic tic pts show higher rates of exacerbations temporally related to strep in PANDAS group, but 75% of exacerbations are not associated.
- Overall 0.56 exacerbations per pt-yr.

Pathophys

- No identified specific anti-neuronal autoimmune antibody marker

Lab

- Look for and treat source of strep.
- ASO and anti-DNAse B titers.

Rx

- Treatment indicated if antibody positive even if surface swabs negative. Use of plasmapheresis as well as IVIg has shown some benefit in research studies but not ready for general use.

4.18 Infantile Botulism

General Ref

- *NEJM* 2006;354(5):462–471
- *Pediatrics* 1991;87:159

Def

- Neurologic impairment caused by activation of *C. botulinum* spores in gi tract of infants; in United States, typically type A or B toxin

Epidem

- More common in areas where soil is disrupted (farming, new development) and rare in inner city. Breastfeeding is risk factor, perhaps related to stool pH and altered flora. Can occur up to 11 months in breastfed infants; formula-fed infants usually < 2 months of age. Constipation is both risk factor and symptom. Younger infants have more severe course.

Pathophys

- Endogenous flora fails to competitively inhibit the activation of spores. Botulinum toxin inhibits Ach release; descending paresis over hours to days, beginning with cranial nerves to upper extremities/trunk/lower extremities.

Clinical Findings

- Constipation, weak suck, floppiness, weak cry, ptosis, head lag, difficulty swallowing. Half have sluggish pupil responses. Asymmetric neurologic impairment, lack of cranial nerve involvement, or an ascending pattern r/o infant botulism.

Diff Dx

- May misdiagnose as septic, but usually have no fever/hematologic abnormalities, mottling. Consider Guillain-Barré, tick paralysis, hypothyroidism, and myasthenia.

Lab

- Mouse assay for toxin. EMG (not typical) has specific pattern.

Rx

- Botulinum immune globulin (BabyBIG-IV) has cut by more than half the duration of intubation, hospitalization, ICU care, and tube feeding for typical case. Still on ventilator for almost 2 wk. Best if given within 72 hr. ICU care to prevent AOM, aspiration pneumonia, catheter-related UTIs, IV line infections, and *C. difficile*.

Chapter 5
Gastroenterology

5.1 Encopresis

General Ref

- *Arch Dis Child* 2007;92:486
- *J Pediatr Gastroenterol Nutr* 2007;44:5–13

Def

- Passage of stool in inappropriate places after the age of 4 yr; may be voluntary or involuntary, with no organic cause

Cause

- Diet, constipation and functional fecal retention, colon lesions, hypothyroidism, autonomic neuropathies

Epidem

- M:F: 2–6:1

Pathophys

- Retention, chronic constipation, fecal impaction resulting in overflow incontinence.
- Rectal distention results in reduced sensation.
- Potential triggers to retention: fissures/painful defecation, reluctance to use school bathrooms, difficult toilet training.
- In most cases no cause found.

S + S

- Abdominal cramps, decreased appetite, secondary daytime enuresis common, 40% fecal mass palpable, normal or decreased sphincter tone, large diameter bowel movements that obstruct the toilet not uncommon.

Course

- Complications: fecal impaction, social problems, UTI, enuresis, decreased appetite

Lab

- No labs needed if hx clear

Xray

- Plain abdominal Xray.
- Atypical findings suggestive of neurologic problem such as tethered chord: consider MRI.

Rx

- Behavioral modification: sit on toilet for 5–10 min once or twice a day after a meal; feet should be firmly balanced on the ground, not hanging; positive motivation; avoid stress around toilet training. Follow-up monthly to ensure compliance and help motivation.
- Dietary changes: high fiber, increase fluid intake.
- Medication often needed for > 6 months: continue until diet and behavior modified and rectal distention resolved. Stool softeners such as milk of magnesia 0.5–1 mL/kg per day, MiraLAX 0.75 mg/kg per day, mineral oil + stimulant laxative senna or docusate. Avoid enemas in toddlers.
- Referral to gastroenterologist for anorectal manometry for pts with recalcitrant sx.

5.2   Pyloric Stenosis

General Ref

- *Arch Pediatr Adolesc Med* 2005;159:520
- *BMJ* 1993;27:306

Cause

- Likely multifactorial inheritance

Epidem

- 1 in 600
- M:F: 4:1
- More common in whites
- More common if maternal family hx

Pathophys

- Concentric hypertrophy of pyloric smooth muscle precipitated by nitric oxide synthetase deficiency (*N Engl J Med* 1992;327:511)

S+S

- Nonbilious projectile vomiting for 2–8 wk in otherwise healthy, hungry baby; weight loss; dehydration in 70%; olive (mass) in RUQ; visible peristalsis after a feed

Course

- Low morbidity and mortality

Complications

- Dehydration, electrolyte abnormalities

Lab

- Metabolic panel, hypochloremic, hypokalemic, alkalosis, hyponatremia with paradoxical aciduria

Xray

- US confirms dx; UGI endoscopy may differentiate other obstructive lesions (e.g., antral webs).

Rx

- Correct electrolyte abnormalities; pyloromyotomy (Ramstedt procedure).

5.3   Gluten Enteropathy: Celiac Disease

General Ref

- *N Engl J Med* 2002;346;180
- *J Pediatr* 2005;40:1–19, gastroenterology and nutrition

Cause

- Genetic component: association with DQ2 and DQ8; not all pts with these markers will get celiac disease (CD), but those who are negative for these markers are very unlikely to develop CD.
- Increased incidence in these conditions: Down syndrome, DM 1, Turner syndrome, Williams syndrome, IgA deficiency, Hashimoto thyroiditis.

Epidem

- Prevalence 1% in United States.
- Primarily affects whites.
- Associated with dermatitis herpetiformis, an itchy skin rash; improves on a gluten-free diet.

Pathophys

- Immune-mediated enteropathy.

- T-cell and IgA-mediated immune response to gluten in genetically predisposed individuals.
- Malabsorption and GI bleeding lead to IDA.

S+S

- Wide range of presentations:
  - Gi manifestation: diarrhea with failure to thrive, abdominal pain and distension, vomiting, constipation
  - Non-gi manifestations: dermatitis herpetiformis (resolves with a gluten-free diet); delayed puberty, osteoporosis, IDA nonresponsive to oral iron treatment

Course

- Normal prognosis on gluten-free diet

Complications

- Short stature, increased incidence of tumors of esophagus and stomach and lymphoma, fertility problems, behavioral problems

Lab

- Endoscopic biopsy of duodenum shows subvillous atrophy and crypt hyperplasia.
- Antiendomysial antibody, antigliadin antibody (used less frequently; other 2 antibodies better); tissue transglutaminase antibody.
- HLA and genetic screening (not routine: helpful with dx dilemmas).
- CBC: mixed anemia.
- Hypocalcemia.
- Increased alkaline phosphatase; mild elevations of AST and ALT.

Xray

- Small bowel followthrough

Rx

- Gluten-free diet for life
- Benefits of treatment: resolve sx of diarrhea and poor weight gain and reverse reduced bone mineralization

5.4 Milk Protein Sensitivity

General Ref

- *Pediatr Allergy Immunol* 1994;1–36
- *Ann Allergy Asthma Immunol* 2002;89:56–60

Cause

- More common with family hx of atopy, with early milk protein–based formulas and with gi infections

Epidem

- 2–7.5% of otherwise normal infants; dx usually < 2 yr

Pathophys

- Immune response to proteins in the whey fraction (unprocessed cow's milk 80% casein and 19% whey; ≥ 20 antigenic proteins in the whey fraction)
- Formation of circulating IgG antibodies and mucosal IgA antibodies, which are thought to be protective
- May also occur in exclusively breast-fed babies through exposure to allergens appearing in breast milk

S+S

- Blood and mucus in stool: common presenting complaint in otherwise normal child.
- Sx resolve with removal of cow's milk protein.

- May not resolve with soy-based formula and may need hydrolyzed formula.
- FTT, vomiting, diarrhea, abdominal distention, stool positive for occult blood.

Course

- Benign with removal of cow's milk proteins

Lab

- CBC: may be eosinophilia, hypoproteinemia
- Stool cultures to r/o infective cause
- Rectosigmoid biopsy: not done routinely; nonspecific changes in bowel mucosa

Rx

- Removal of products containing cow's milk protein usually causes resolution of bloody diarrhea in 24–72 hr although may remain guaiac positive for 2–6 wk.
- Usually tolerance to cow's milk protein by 1 yr of age and can be safely reintroduced.
- 10% may persist to 6 yr.

5.5 Food Allergies

General Ref

- *Pediatrics* 2003;111(6), supplement on food allergy
- *Pediatric Ann* 37(8), update on food allergy
- *Pediatrics* 121(1), Committee on Nutrition

Def

- Immunologically mediated pathologic response caused by exposure to food antigens. Classic allergic reactions are IgE mediated, but the term *food allergy* includes non-IgE or mixed reactions. Food intolerances are due to nonimmune mechanisms, such as malabsorption of food components (lactose, fat, etc.) or idiosyncratic reactions to natural or artificial chemicals in foods (tyramine, caffeine).

Sx

- *Anaphylaxis*: oral tingling, swelling of lips, followed by nausea/pain/vomiting/diarrhea; typically associated with flushing or urticaria; laryngeal swelling and stridor may follow, or bronchospasm; lightheadedness can progress to syncope or hypotension.
- Milder IgE-mediated reactions involve only urticaria/angioedema or just rhinitis.
- *Oral allergy syndrome*: mild local pruritus limited to mouth area due to cross sensitivity between food allergens and some pollens. Raw foods trigger reactions, but cooked foods usually are tolerated.
- *Eczema*: thought to be mixture of IgE and non-IgE mechanism. Food is significant trigger in one-third of children (milk, egg, peanut).
- *Eosinophilic esophagitis* mimics severe reflux with FTT, vomiting, dysphagia, abdominal pain, protein-losing enteropathy (if more generalized).
- *Proctocolitis* considered non-IgE mechanism. Hematochezia in healthy breast or formula-fed infant. Restrictions from milk and soy protein for 1st yr of life resolves.
- A more serious version of *food protein-induced enterocolitis* presents as recurrent vomiting, diarrhea, anemia, and FTT. Milk and soy protein most common, and *not* IgE mediated; skin testing not useful; rice and other cereals, meats, and so on can also trigger.

Epidem

- 1–200 deaths per year. All ages, but two-thirds between age 13–21 yr because they eat more away from home, more risk taking.

- Peanut, tree nut, fish/shellfish are predominant foods.
- Hx asthma is risk factor for deaths. Reactions can be biphasic: initial phase, 3–30 min and second phase 20–150 min. Severity of prior reaction not predictive.
- Overall prevalence of food allergy varies with strictness of definition. Milk allergy tends to wane with age; peanut and tree nut allergies tend to persist.

Dx

- Based on detailed hx of events—portion size, sequence and timing of sx, consistency of reactions from event to event, other possible foods. Physical exam looks for evidence of allergy in general: nasal, respiratory, skin. Use of elimination diets can guide therapy if specific food likely (*Pediatrics* 101(6):1640), but more general elimination diets can lead to malnutrition. Skin testing has a high negative predictive value, but positive responses need clinical correlation. RAST testing. Non-IgE illness can be diagnosed with endoscopy/biopsy and/or elimination diets.

Rx

- Avoidance of offending antigen. For milk allergy, breastfeeding with maternal restriction, or, in formula-fed infants, use of hydrolyzed hypoallergenic formula (Nutramigen, Alimentum). Rarely, more aggressively hydrolyzed formula needed (Neocate, EleCare, or Nutramigen AA).
- Timely administration of epinephrine via an autoinjector prevents progression of anaphylactic sx and should be delivered if any hives, respiratory sx, oral thickening, vomiting, or hypotension. Antihistamines and steroids can be useful adjuncts.
- For non-IgE food reactions, there is limited data to support the use of oral cromolyn, topical or systemic steroids, leukotriene inhibitors, or probiotics.

5.6 Diarrhea

General Ref

- *N Engl J Med* 2006;355:236
- *Pediatr Rev* 1998;19:418–422

5.6.1 Microvillous Inclusion Disease

Cause

- Autosomal recessive

S+S

- Most common cause of persistent diarrhea in the neonatal period
- Presents with intractable diarrhea and malabsorption in the neonatal period

Rx

- Long-term TPN; intestinal transplant

5.6.2 Glucose-Galactose Malabsorption

Cause

- Rare autosomal recessive disorder

S+S

- Rapid onset of watery diarrhea from birth
- Responds to withholding glucose; relapse if reintroduced

Lab

- Clinical dx
- Stool positive for reducing substances
- Small intestinal biopsy is normal

Rx

- Substitute fructose for glucose as the main carbohydrate source.
- Fructose is absorbed by a different mechanism than glucose and galactose.

5.6.3 Congenital Intestinal Lymphangiectasia

Cause

- Functional obstruction of lymphatic flow from thoracic duct to inferior vena cava

Epidem

- Occurs in infancy and childhood

S+S

- Malabsorption, diarrhea, nausea, vomiting, abdominal pain

Lab

- Low calcium, protein, and albumin
- Decreased immunoglobulins
- Decreased lymphocytes

Rx

- Medium-chain triglycerides; low-fat, high-protein diet

5.6.4 Toddler's Diarrhea

General Ref

- *Pediatr Clin North Am* 1996;43:375–390
- *J Pediatr Gastroenterol Nutr* 1985;4:362–365

Cause

- Also called chronic nonspecific diarrhea

Epidem

- Most common cause of persistent loose stool in preschool children

Pathophys

- Underlying maturational delay in intestinal motility

S + S

- Well-formed to very loose stools; undigested vegetables often present; child otherwise well and thriving with no obvious dietary triggers to sx

Course

- Most children grow out of sx by 5 yr

Rx

- No treatment required.
- Consider cautious use of loperamide in socially disruptive sx.

5.7   Inflammatory Bowel Disease

- The idiopathic inflammatory bowel diseases (IBDs) include CD and UC. Evidence suggests that IBD results from an inappropriate inflammatory response to intestinal microbes in a genetically susceptible host. Genetic studies highlight the importance of host–microbe interactions in the pathogenesis of these diseases.

5.7.1 Crohn's Disease

General Ref

- *N Engl J Med* 2009;361:2066–2078
- *Cochrane Database Syst Rev* 2003;(4):CD000301

Cause

- Unknown

Epidem

- Worldwide incidence increasing since the 1950s
- Progressively more common throughout childhood
- 4.56 per 100,000 population
- M:F: 1:1; bimodal age of onset with peaks in the 20s–30s and in the 60s
- 2% before age 10 yr

Pathophys

- Discrete areas of focal ulceration with normal intervening mucosa. CD is a transmural, focal, subacute, and chronic inflammatory disease. It may affect the gi tract from mouth to anus. Hallmark of the disease is the presence of noncaseating epithelioid cell granulomata.

S+S

- Presentation depends on location and extent of inflammation.
- Common presenting features include abdominal pain, diarrhea, fever, weight loss, growth failure, oral and perianal ulcers.
- Extraintestinal sx: erythema nodosum, pyoderma gangrenosum, anemia, hepatitis, nephrolithiasis, arthritis, clubbing, malaise, anorexia, uveitis, delayed puberty.

Course

- Long-term prognosis good, in general, with most pts leading normal lives despite occasional recurrences

Complications

- Strictures, fistulas, abscesses, malabsorption, small bowel obstruction, growth failure. Surgery may be required.

Lab

- Colonoscopy, biopsy, and histology: characteristic noncaseating granuloma.
- Acute phase reactants: ESR and CRP are usually elevated and can be used to monitor disease severity.

Xray

- Barium followthrough: characteristic narrowing, fissures, mucosal irregularities, and mural thickening

Rx

- Goal: to induce remission by suppressing inflammation.
- No drug regimens have been found to alter long-term outcome of CD.
- Remission: 5-aminosalicylic acid preparations, folate supplements
- Acute exacerbations: mesalamine 30–60 mg/kg per day divided in 3–4 doses; mesalamine enemas daily for distal colitis, methylprednisone or prednisone: 1–2 mg/kg per day in 2 divided doses. Taper and discontinue once remission is achieved.
- Perianal disease or fistulas: metronidazole 15 mg/kg per day in 3 divided doses; ciprofloxacin 250–500 mg twice a day.
- Refractory disease:
  - Azathioprine 2–3mg/kg per day in 2 divided doses
  - 6 mercaptopurine 1–2mg/kg per day in 2 divided doses
  - Methotrexate 15 mg sc or im weekly
  - Infliximab 5 mg/kg IV infusion over 2 hr at wk 0, 2, and 6 (*Lancet* 2002;359:1541; *J Pediatr* 2000;137:192–196)

5.7.2 Ulcerative Colitis

General Ref

- *Gastroenterology* 2007;133:423–432
- *J Pediatr Gastroenterol Nutr* 1999;28:54–58

Cause

- Unknown; genetic immunologic factors implicated.
- No specific heritable pattern but 15–40% will have a family hx of IBD.

Epidem

- General population incidence 4.1–7.3 per 100,000
- Incidence 10–19 yr of age, 2–4 per 100,000
- More common in whites 2F:1M
- 15–40% present < 20 yr with 10% presenting < 10 yr, although rare younger than 2 yr

Pathophys

- Recurrent, inflammatory, ulcerating disease involving submucosal and mucosal infiltration by polymorphonuclear leukocytes and mononuclear cells, rarely extending beyond the muscularis mucosa; limited to colon and rectum

S+S

- Diarrhea, abdominal pain, urgency, weight loss, anorexia, fever. In severe disease may be more than 6 bloody stools per day.
- Extraintestinal: erythema nodosum, pyoderma gangrenosum, arthritis and spondylitis, cholangitis.

Course

- 80% recur within 1 yr; 100% within 17 yr.

Complications

- Toxic megacolon in ≤ 5%: a surgical and medical emergency with associated risk of perforation, gram-negative sepsis, and massive hemorrhage

- Increased incidence of adenocarcinoma of the colon in adulthood (1 in 200 risk for each yr of disease between 10 and 20 yr from dx)
- Hepatitis, sclerosing cholangitis

Lab

- CBC shows leucocytosis and anemia.
- Acute phase reactants: elevated.
- Low serum protein, albumin, iron, zinc, and magnesium.
- Electrolyte disturbances uncommon unless dehydrated.
- Stool to r/o infectious colitis.
- Colonoscopy and histology characteristic features (barium enema no longer recommended as a screening procedure because colonoscopy has greater diagnostic value).
- Wireless capsule endoscopy may be validated and adapted to pediatrics in the future.

Rx

- Mild disease: disease localized to distal colon and maintenance therapy:
  - Sulfasalazine 50–75 mg/kg per day in 2–3 divided doses
  - 5-ASA 30–80 mg/kg per day po, enema, or suppository
  - Daily folic acid 1 mg/day
- Moderate to severe disease:
  - Hospitalize.
  - Broad-spectrum antibiotics.
  - Methylprednisone 1–2 mg/kg per day in 2 divided doses for 2 wk; then taper dose and discontinue once remission is established.
  - Sulfasalazine 40–50 mg/kg per day in 2–3 divided doses; gradually increase dose to a maximum of 3–4 g per day during steroid taper.
  - Folate 1 mg/kg per day.

- Refractory disease (*J Pediatr Gastroenterol Nutr* 1999;28:54–58):
  - Azathioprine 2–2.5 mg/kg per day
  - 6 mercaptopurine 1–1.5 mg/kg per day

5.8   Chronic Hepatitis

General Ref

- *J Pediatr Gastroenterol Nutr* 2002;35:S39
- *Mod Pathol* 1994;7:690

Cause

- May occur due to persistent hepatic viral infection with hepatitis B, D, and C due to chronic autoimmune hepatitis or due to drugs

Epidem

- High incidence in Southeast Asia, China, and Africa; affects perinatal and preschool ages in endemic areas, adolescents elsewhere

Pathophys

Damage to the hepatocytes with infiltration of inflammatory cells and liver regeneration. Depending on the typical pathological findings, classified as chronic persistent hepatitis, chronic aggressive hepatitis, or chronic lobular hepatitis.

S+S

- Insidious onset with fatigue, fever, abdominal pain, nausea, diarrhoea, anorexia, depression, jaundice. Pediatric pts with autoimmune hepatitis may have an acute onset of sx.

Course

- Depends on the cause, but many will go on to end stage liver disease requiring liver transplant.

Lab

- CBC, LFTs, serum proteins, serum immunoglobulins.
- Liver bx needed to make the dx. Characteristic pathologic findings will be specific to the cause (e.g., ground-glass appearance in chronic hepatitis B, fatty infiltration in chronic hepatitis C).

Rx

- Specific treatment is that of the underlying cause.
- General treatment:
  - Ensure immunizations up-to-date including hepatitis A
  - Maintain adequate nutrition: supplement fat soluble vitamins D, A, K and E, aggressive weight management if NASH (non-alcoholic steatohepatitis) due to obesity and the metabolic syndrome
  - Treat pruritis with antihistamines, cholesytramine, naltrexone, or rifampicin
  - Aggressively treat spontaneous bacterial peritonitis (SBP)
  - Address psychosocial aspect with referral to counselor, clinical psychologists
  - Early referral to liver transplant center

5.9 Viral Hepatitis

5.9.1 Hepatitis A

General Ref

- *Pediatr Rev* 2001;22:219
- *Clin Liver Dis* 2006;10:27

Cause

- A single-stranded RNA enterovirus

Epidem

- Transmission usually fecal oral; incidence has fallen with improved socioeconomic conditions; incubation period 15–40 d.

Pathophys

- Liver inflammation and necrosis

S+S

- Asymptomatic to mild sx in children

Course

- Recovery within 2–4 wk; do not develop chronic liver disease

Lab

- Anti-HAV IgM

Rx

- No treatment; self-limiting
- Prophylaxis for close contacts with human immunoglobulin or vaccinated within 2 wk of onset of illness

5.9.2 Hepatitis B

General Ref

- *J Gastroenterol Hepatol* 2004;19:127–133
- *Eur J Pediatr* 1998;157:382–385

Cause

- A hepadnavirus

Epidem

- Incubation period 50–150 d
- Children affected through vertical transmission, blood, and blood products
- Sexual transmission in adolescents

S+S

- Children, especially infants, may be asymptomatic; fever, jaundice, dark urine, pale stools. Infants infected by vertical transmission usually become asymptomatic carriers.

Course

- Most resolve spontaneously.
- 1–2% develop fulminant hepatic failure.
- 5–10% become chronic carriers; of these carriers, 30–50% develop chronic HBV liver disease; 10% of these may develop cirrhosis.

Complications

- Glomerulonephritis or nephrotic syndrome due to immune complexes, cirrhosis, and hepatocellular carcinoma

Lab

- HBsAg, anti-HBc IgM confirm infection.
- HBeAg persistence is a marker of infectivity.
- Anti-HBe implies termination of viral replication.
- HbsAg confirms vertical infection.
- Anti-HBc indicates previous infection.
- Anti-HBs signifies recovery, immunity, or response to vaccine.
- HBsAg persists > 8 wk in chronic infection (by definition chronic infection lasts > 6 months).
- LFTs: elevated aminotransferases, conjugated and unconjugated bilirubin; normal to low WCC; elevated ESR

Rx

- Prevention:
  - If mother HBsAg positive, baby is given hepatitis B vaccine at birth; also given IVIG if mother also HBeAg positive.
    - Supportive treatment in acute hepatitis B infection
    - Chronic hepatitis B: interferon alpha 5–6 million units/m² body surface area sc 3 times daily for 4–6 wk.
    - Lamivudine 3 mg/kg per day to maximum 100 mg daily for 12 months; limited by development of resistance.
    - Newer drugs such as adefovir or long-acting (pegylated) interferon: promising results in children.

5.9.3 Hepatitis C

General Ref

- *Red Book*: 2009 Report of the Committee on Infectious Diseases
- *Hepatology* 2005;42:1010–1018

Cause

- RNA flavivirus

Epidem

- Transmission vertical, parenteral, or sexual; incubation period 30–150 d. Prevalence in the United States 0.6%; higher in IV drug users. Vertical transmission rare unless coinfection with HIV and associated with viremia.

Pathophys

- Changes in the liver include steatosis, sinusoidal lymphocytosis, portal lymphoid aggregates.

S+S

- Mild or asymptomatic; often incidental finding of elevated aminotransferases

Course

- Acute infection rare; 50% develop chronic liver disease.

Complications

- Cirrhosis and hepatocellular carcinoma after several years

Lab

- Anti-HCV, PCR RNA
- Infants born to HCV-positive mothers may have persistence of maternal antibodies for 18 months. In this case, check HCV PCR at 6 wk and 6 months: positive at 6 months presumed infected, negative at 6 months follow labs to document clearance of HCV antibodies.

Rx

- Combination of interferon or peginterferon and ribavirin effective in 50% of children

5.9.4 Hepatitis D

General Ref

- *Curr Top Microbiol Immunol* 2006;307:151–171

Cause

- Defective RNA virus that depends on hepatitis B for replication

Epidem

- Transmitted parenterally and sexually; incubation period 20–90 d; risk factors as for those for HBV infection

Pathophys

- Virion particle enclosing HDV RNA is encased within HBsAg coat.

S+S

- Usually mild, self-limiting infection. Chronic carriers of HBV who become superinfected with HDV may result in increased disease severity.

Course

- Cirrhosis develops in 50–70% of those with chronic HDV infection.

Complications

- Fulminant hepatitis

Lab

- Anti-HDV

Rx

- Supportive measures; no specific treatment is available.
- Treatment and prevention of HBV.

5.9.5 Hepatitis E

General Ref

- *Proc Natl Acad Sci USA* 2009;106:12992–12997
- *J Gastroenterol Hepatol* 2004;19:778–784

Cause

- RNA calicivirus

Epidem

- Fecal oral transmission; incubation period 15–40 d; epidemics occur in some developing countries; 10% mortality in pregnant women

S+S

- Mild to severe sx

Course

- No evidence of chronic infection

Lab

- Serologic assays for HEV

Rx

- No treatment currently available; trials in progress to develop a recombinant vaccine

5.10   Pancreatitis

General Ref

- *N Engl J Med* 2006;354:2142
- *Am J Gastroenterol* 2002;97:1726

Cause

- Acute and chronic inflammation of the pancreas. Causes include idiopathic; infections such as typhoid, mycoplasma; virus: coxsackie B, EBV; hyperlipidemia; hypercalcemia; drugs; toxins; autoimmune; structural anomalies of the pancreas.

Pathophys

- Stasis in the pancreatic duct leading to cytokine release and activation of pancreatic proenzymes. Familial pancreatitis due to mutation in the following genes:
  - Cationic trypsinogen gene enhances trypsin activity (e.g., PRSS1).
  - SPINK1, serine protease inhibitor Kazal type 1 gene resulting in abnormal pancreatic secretory trypsin inhibitor.
  - CFTR, CF transmembrane conductance regulator gene, which reduces the pancreatic fluid secretion capacity; increased risk of keeping activated trypsin I in the pancreas for a longer period.

S+S

- Acute:
  - Anorexia, nausea, vomiting, fever, epigastric pain radiating to the back, with some relief by leaning forward, and aggravation by food.
  - Presentations range from mild to hypotension and shock.
  - Retroperitoneal hemorrhage manifest as Cullen sign: periumbilical ecchymosis; Grey Turner: flank ecchymosis.
- Chronic:
  - Vomiting, chronic epigastric abdominal pain radiating to the back, aggravated by food, repeated acute episodes
  - Loose foul-smelling stools due to protein and fat malabsorption, FTT, glucose intolerance, and DM

Course

- Depends on the severity at presentation.
- Adult severity scores have not been validated in children (Ransom, APACHE).
- Worse prognosis if present with hypotension, shock, renal failure, pulmonary edema.

Lab

- CBC, metabolic panel, LFTs, amylase, lipase, low fecal elastase
- Genetic testing for PRSS1, SPINK1, CFTR if a family hx of hereditary pancreatitis or hx of recurrent acute or unexplained chronic pancreatitis

Imaging

- Abdominal ultrasound may show enlarged pancreas, dilated ducts, pseudocyst, and gallbladder.
- Abdominal CT: may show hemorrhage, necrosis, pseudocysts.
- ERCP: sensitive and specific for choledochal cysts and divisum.

Rx

- NPO, IV fluid resuscitation.
- Pain management with morphine or meperidine.
- Start enteral feeds once pain subsides (*BMJ* 2004;328:1407).
- Antibiotics reserved for severe cases with necrotizing disease.
- ERCP sphincterotomy.
- US-guided aspiration of pseudocysts.
- Considerations in chronic pancreatitis:
  - Treatment as above; in addition:
    - Low-fat diet and pancreatic enzyme replacement.
    - Islet cell autotransplantation: total pancreatectomy followed by reimplantation of islet cells into liver; may improve glycemic control and pain.

5.11   Gastroesophageal Reflux

General Ref

- *J Pediatr Gastroenterol Nutr* 2001;32:S1–31

Cause

- Acidity from reflux of stomach contents for > 4% of the time in a 24-hr period (normal individuals should be for < 4%).

Epidem

- Occurs in otherwise normal infants with increased risk in cerebral palsy, premature babies, and following surgery for esophageal atresia or diaphragmatic hernia

Pathophys

- Short intra-abdominal length of esophagus and functional immaturity of the lower esophageal sphincter leading to episodes of inappropriate relaxation

S+S

- May present with frequent regurgitation

Course

- Common in 1st yr of life; usually resolves spontaneously by 1 yr.

Complications

- IDA, apnea, apparent life-threatening events, dystonic movements of head and neck

Lab

- 24-hr esophageal pH study
- Endoscopy with biopsy if esophagitis is suspected

Rx

- Mild reflux: thickening of feeds, positioning in 30° head up; prone position after feeds.

- More severe reflux: proton pump inhibitors (e.g., omeprazole to reduce esophagitis; drugs that enhance gastric emptying, e.g., domperidone).
- Severe refractory reflux with complications such as esophageal strictures or recurrent respiratory sx and aspiration may be considered for surgical intervention: fundoplication.

5.12 Recurrent Abdominal Pain

General Ref

- *Pediatrics* 2005;115:812–815
- *Am J Gastroenterol* 2005;100:1868–1875

Def

- Recurrent pain sufficient to interrupt normal activity lasting at least 3 months

Cause

- Less than 10% have definable organic cause.

Epidem

- Common; affects up to 10% of school-age children, girls more than boys; family hx is common, usually periumbilical.

Pathophys

- May be a manifestation of stress. There is evidence that anxiety may lead to altered gi motility, which may be perceived as pain.

S+S

- A prolonged hx is not a risk factor for an organic cause.
- Red flags suggesting organic origin include diarrhea, vomiting weight loss, FTT, joint sx, fever, blood in stool, nighttime pain.

Course

- 50% rapidly become sx free; 25% take months to resolve; 25% continue or return in adulthood as IBS, nonulcer dyspepsia, or cranial migraine.

Lab

- Urine microscopy and culture
- CBC
- Inflammatory markers and celiac screen

Rx

- Reassurance

5.13   Acute Abdomen

General Ref

- *Emerg Med Clin North Am* 2002;20:139–153

Diff Dx

- Intestinal problems (e.g., gastroenteritis, acute appendicitis, PUD, intestinal obstruction)
- Pancreatic conditions (e.g., pancreatitis)
- Hepatobiliary conditions (e.g., hepatitis, Wilson disease, hepatic tumor)
- Genitourinary conditions (e.g., pyelonephritis, ovarian conditions, testicular torsion)
- Systemic conditions (e.g., DKA, porphyria)

Cause

- Surgical causes to exclude in childhood acute abdominal pain:
  - Infancy:
    - Volvulus, stenosis, duplications, incarcerated hernias, testicular torsion, Meckel diverticulum, obstruction

with or without ischemia, intussusception, appendicitis, Hirschsprung disease
- Children
  - Perforation, blunt trauma, ovarian lesion, foreign body, neoplasia, Meckel diverticulum, intussusception, appendicitis

5.13.1 Appendicitis

General Ref

- *Surg Infect* 2004;5:349–356

Cause

- Acute inflammation of the appendix

Epidem

- Most common cause of abdominal pain in childhood requiring surgical intervention
- Rare in infancy

S+S

- Vomiting, anorexia, low-grade fever, acute abdominal pain and guarding, may be diarrhea but not usually as severe as in gastroenteritis.
- In early pelvic appendicitis there may be no abdomen pain but severe rectal tenderness.

Course

- Recovery usually rapid with excellent prognosis if no perforation. Perforation more common in children due to delay in dx.

Lab

- CBC; elevated WCC with left shift

Imaging

- Abdominal Xray may be normal; may show a calcified fecalith.
- Abdominal US: edema, inflammation, abscess formation.
- Abdominal CT.

Rx

- IV fluids, correct electrolyte imbalances, nasogastric tube.
- Broad-spectrum antibiotics and pain medication.
- Emergency appendectomy: laparoscopic appendectomy associated with earlier recovery (*Ann Surg* 2006;243: 17–27; *Cochrane Database Syst Rev* 2004;(4): CD001546).

5.13.2 Hirschsprung Disease

General Ref

- *Am J Surg* 2000;180:382

Cause

- Abnormal innervation of the distal bowel

Epidem

- Most common cause of lower intestinal obstruction in neonates.
- 5% of pts with Hirschsprung disease have mutations in the endothelin signaling pathway.
- M:F: 1:4

Pathophys

- Absence of Meissner and Auerbach plexuses starting from rectum extending proximally for variable lengths

S + S

- Failure to pass meconium by 48 hr of life, delayed passage of meconium, abdominal distention, bilious vomiting, small-volume stools

Lab

- CBC: anemia and leucocytosis
- Anorectal manometry (ARM)
- Rectal suction biopsy diagnostic (RSB)
- ARM and RSB found to be most accurate tests in diagnostic workup (*J Pediatr Gastroenterol Nutr* 2006;42:496–505)

Imaging

- Plain abdominal film: may show distended loops of bowel
- Barium contrast enema

Rx

- IV fluids, nasogastric tube
- Broad-spectrum antibiotics
- Definitive treatment: surgical excision of affected segments usually involving an initial colostomy followed by anastomosis of normal bowel to anus

5.13.3 Intussusception

General Ref

- *Am J Emerg* 1997;15:293
- *Pediatrics* 2007;120:473

Cause

- Invagination of proximal bowel into a distal segment; usually no underlying cause

Epidem

- Most common abdominal emergency in early childhood
- M:F: 3:2
- Peak age: 2 months to 2 yr
- 90% ileocolic type
- Associated with rotavirus and Henoch-Schönlein purpura

S+S

- Paroxysmal colicky abdominal pain and pallor, well between episodes, palpable sausage-shaped mass in abdomen, red currant jelly stool

Course

- Good outcome if diagnosed early; 10% recurrence after non-operative reduction

Complications

- Gi bleeding, perforation, sepsis, shock

Lab

- CBC, metabolic panel

Xray

- Plain abdominal Xray: distend loops of small bowel, absence of gas in distal colon and rectum, air fluid levels
- Abdominal US (*Pediatr Radiol* 2009;39:1075): for dx and assessing success of reduction
- Barium enema

Rx

- Nasogastric tube to decompress bowel.
- IV fluids; correct electrolyte imbalance.

- Reduction via barium enema (contraindicated if peritonitis, shock, or perforation).
- Failed reduction surgical correction.

Chapter 6
Nephrology

6.1 Nephrotic Syndrome

General Ref

- *Nephrol Dial Transplant* 2003;18:vi, 75
- *Pediatr Nephrol* 2004;19:281

Cause

- Congenital nephrotic syndrome (NS): rare autosomal recessive form of congenital NS due to mutation in nephrin gene NPHS1.
- Presents with edema as early as day 2 of life, associated with a large placenta, resistant to steroid therapy, usually need kidney transplant once pt has reached 10 kg (*Pediatr Nephrol* 2003;18:426; *Curr Opin Pediatr* 2004;16:165).
- Primary NS can occur in any of the childhood glomerulonephritides:
  - Minimal-change glomerulonephritis (MCGN) most common, the cause in 76% of children and 20% of adults
  - Membranous GN the cause in 7% of children and 40% of adults
  - Diffuse mesangial proliferative cause in 4% of children and 7% of adults
  - Focal segmental glomerulosclerosis (FSGS): increasing incidence in pediatric population of 15–25% (previously

around 8%); cause for the increase unknown; the cause in 15% of adults
- Membranoproliferative GN 5% of children and 18% of adults
- Secondary NS:
  - Other renal disease (e.g., IgA nephropathy, hemolytic uremic syndrome)
  - Familial disorders (e.g., Alport syndrome, congenital NS, Fabry's disease)
  - Medications (e.g., penicillamine, gold, chronic IV heroin use) (*N Engl J Med* 1974;290:19)
  - Infections (e.g., bacterial, viral, parasitic)
  - Malignancies (e.g., Wilms tumor, leukemia, lymphoma)
  - Systemic disorders (e.g., SLE and other collagen vascular diseases; sarcoidosis)
  - Allergic reactions (e.g., insect stings, snake venom, serum sickness)

Epidem

- Annual incidence 2–4 cases per 100,000 children < 19 yr; M:F: 3:2

Pathophys

- Changes in glomerular barrier result in protein loss in urine.
- Three mechanisms identified:
  - Loss of negative charge along GBM (glomerular basement membrane) and epithelial surface without structural damage. Electron microscopy shows small cavities of uniform size scattered throughout GBM. This is the mechanism in MCGN.
  - Separation of epithelial podocytes from GBM; most common mechanism in FSGS. Genetic mutations in

glomerular podocyte proteins may predispose some children to FSGS.
- Appearance of gaps in GBM through which blood and cells may pass.

S+S

- Sx: periorbital edema in the morning, pedal edema later in the day, often preceding influenza-like syndrome, malaise, occasional abdominal discomfort
- Si: edema, anasarca, dyspnea due to pleural effusions

Course

- Secondary causes may reverse after treatment of primary cause.
- Minimal change NS, occurring between 1 and 10 yr: > 90% steroid responsive.
- Prognosis poorer in the following situations:
  - Pt < 1 yr or > 10 yr, persistent hematuria, hypertension, renal failure, failure to respond to steroids within 4 wk
- In the situations just described, bx is indicated. The histologic type determines clinical outcome more than any other factor.

Complications

- Infections (e.g., peritonitis)
- Hyperlipidemia
- Hypercoagulability due to loss of ATIII (antithrombin III), protein S, and protein C
- Thromboembolic phenomena due to dehydration and venous stasis
- Hypertension
- Renal failure

Lab

- Proteinuria hallmark of NS
  - Urinalysis: 2–4+ protein dipstick, high specific gravity, hyaline and granular casts
  - Urine 24-hr protein > 3–3.5 g
  - Random urine protein-to-creatinine ratio > 2.0 (normal < 0.2)
  - Low serum albumin
  - Increased serum cholesterol, triglycerides, and total lipids (*Ann Intern Med* 1993;119:263)

Rx

- General measures: sodium restriction.
- ACE inhibitors improve lipids (*Ann Intern Med* 1993;118:246) and lower protein excretion.
- Treat secondary causes.
- Immunizations held until in remission and off steroids for at least 3 months. No live virus vaccine to pt or other household members while pt is taking high-dose steroids or cytotoxic drugs.
- First line:
  - Prednisone 60 mg/m^2 daily for 4 wk, then 40 mg/m^2 alternate days for 4 wk.
  - If no remission with above, nephrology consult.
  - If remission followed by relapse, repeat the course with 60 mg/m^2 daily until remission.
  - Then 40 mg/m^2 daily for 8–12 wk.
- Second line:
  - Frequent relapses (i.e., > 4 per year), consider alternate regimens: levamisole, cyclophosphamide, cyclosporine, tacrolimus, diuretics; careful use as may have decreased circulating volume.

6.2 Renal Tubular Acidosis

6.2.1 Distal Renal Tubular Acidosis Type 1

General Ref

- *Am Soc Nephrol* 2002;13:2160
- *Am Soc Nephrol* 2002;13:2178
- *Clin Pediatr* 2001;40:533

Cause

- Primary causes are sporadic and hereditary:
  - Autosomal dominant (mutation in basolateral Cl^-/HCO_3^- exchanger, AE1 gene located on chromosome 17q21-22)
  - Autosomal recessive with deafness (mutation in B1 subunit of H+-ATPase gene located on chromosome 2p13
  - Autosomal recessive without deafness (mutation in alpha 4 subunit of H+-ATPase gene located on chromosome 7q33-34)
- Secondary causes:
  - Obstructive uropathy, SS, amphotericin and cyclosporine, SLE, rheumatoid arthritis

Pathophys

- Defect in the tubular transport of hydrogen ion in the distal nephron. Impaired distal hydrogen secretion.

S+S

- FTT, hypokalemic weakness, anorexia, vomiting, dehydration

Course

- Genetic types have onset at school age.

Complications

- Nephrocalcinosis, nephrolithiasis, rickets, renal failure

Lab

- Hyperchloremic, normal ion gap metabolic acidosis with hypokalemia is the characteristic finding with these characteristics:
  - Urine pH > 5.8; never acid
  - Hypercalcuria

Rx

- 1–2 mmol/kg per day sodium bicarbonate

6.2.2 Proximal Renal Tubular Acidosis Type 2

Cause

- Isolated defect: sporadic (transient in infancy) and hereditary:
  - Autosomal dominant
  - Autosomal recessive with ocular abnormalities (mutations in Na^+/HCO_3 co-transporter gene located on chromosome 4q21)
- Fanconi syndrome: occurs with several disorders including Lowe syndrome, Wilson disease, cystinosis, tyrosinemia, galactosemia, heavy metal poisoning

Epidem

- Most common form of RTA in childhood

Pathophys

- Impaired proximal tubular HCO_3 reabsorption

S + S

- FTT, vomiting, short stature

Course

- Excellent prognosis in isolated defects. If part of more complex tubule abnormality (e.g., Fanconi syndrome), prognosis depends on underlying disorder.

Complications

- Rarely manifest complications of nephrocalcinosis, nephrolithiasis, or rickets (common in type 1)

Lab

- Hyperchloremic, metabolic acidosis, and hypokalemia
- Hypercalcuria unusual

Rx

- 5–15 mmol/kg per day sodium bicarbonate; larger doses are needed to overcome the low renal threshold.

6.2.3 Hyperkalemic Distal Renal Tubular Acidosis Type 4

Cause

- Aldosterone deficiency: primary: CAH, Addison disease
- Hyporeninemic hypoaldosteronism: diabetic nephropathy, lupus nephropathy, ACEI, COX inhibitors
- Aldosterone resistance: obstructive uropathy, tubulointerstitial nephritis

Pathophys

- Abnormality of distal tubular function of hydrogen and potassium ion handling
- Impaired ammoniagenesis

S+S

- Signs of the primary disorder (e.g., CAH, Addison)

Lab

- Metabolic acidosis, hyponatremia, hyperkalemia, normal renal function

Rx

- 1–5 mmol/kg per day sodium bicarbonate corrects the acidosis and may correct the hyperkalemia.
- May need to use potassium exchange resins to control the potassium; Lasix may also be used but only if no salt wasting.

6.3 Lowe's Syndrome (Oculocerebrorenal Syndrome)

Cause

- X-linked recessive

Pathophys

- Range of mutations in the ORCL1 gene that code for Golgi apparatus phosphatase located on chromosome Xq26.1

S + S

- Typically renal dysfunction in the 1st yr of life in a male pt with congenital cataracts
- Presents in early infancy with congenital cataracts and glaucoma
- Typical facies: epicanthal folds, frontal prominence, scaphocephaly
- Renal tubular dysfunction: Fanconi syndrome
- Mental retardation, muscular hypotonia and areflexia, seizures
- Behavioral problems including stereotypy, temper tantrums; growth failure by 1–3 yr

Course

- Most boys survive to adulthood, surviving adult heights less than 3rd percentile.

Complications

- Hypophosphatemic rickets, chronic renal failure in 2nd to 4th decades of life

Lab

- Proteinuria
- Generalized aminoaciduria in first few months of life
- Low serum phosphorous, low to normal serum calcium, elevated serum alkaline phosphatase
- RTA type 2

Rx

- Symptomatic: alkali therapy, phosphate replacement, vitamin D

6.4 Congenital Hypokalemic Alkalosis

6.4.1 Bartter's Syndrome

General Ref

- *Pediatrics* 2003;112:628
- *Am J Med* 2002;112:3

Cause

- Defect in chloride reabsorption in ascending loop of Henle

Pathophys

- Recessive 3 types:
  - Neonatal Bartter's syndrome (BS) type 1: mutations in the NKCC2 cotransporter gene on chromosome 15q15-21
  - Neonatal BS type 2: mutation ROMK channel gene on chromosome 11q24
  - Classic BS type 3: mutation in the CIC-K channel gene on chromosome 1p36

S+S

- Neonatal BS type 1 and 2: often born prematurely due to severe polyhydramnios, fever, dehydration, recurrent UTI, hypercalcuria with early-onset nephrocalcinosis.

- Classic form (present 6 months to 5 yr): FTT, muscle weakness, polyuria, polydipsia, constipation, short stature, normal BP

Course

- Prognosis guarded
- Neonatal form death from hypokalemia, dehydration, and vascular collapse
- Less severe classic forms compatible with long-term survival

Complications

- Neonatal form: nephrocalcinosis

Lab

- Hypochloremia, hypokalemia, metabolic alkalosis
- Very high circulating renin and aldosterone levels with normal BP
- Normal magnesium
- Elevated PGE2
- Juxtaglomerular hyperplasia on renal biopsy

Rx

- Neonatal BS type 1 and 2: fluid and electrolyte replacement
- Indomethacin 3–5 mg/kg per day divided 3 times per day to correct hyperprostaglandinemia
- Classic BS: prostaglandin inhibitors (e.g., indomethacin, potassium-sparing diuretics, potassium supplements)

6.4.2 Gitelman's Syndrome

General Ref

- *J Am Soc Nephrol* 2007;18:1271–1283

Cause

- Autosomal recessive

Pathophys

- Mutation in NCCT co-transporter gene on chromosome 16q13

S+S

- Diagnosed between 1 and 13 yr; asymptomatic hypokalemia; carpopedal spasm due to hypomagnesemia

Lab

- Hypokalemia, metabolic alkalosis, hypochloremia, hypomagnesemia, hypocalciuria; increased renin and aldosterone

Rx

- High doses potassium and magnesium; potassium-sparing diuretics

6.5 Glomerular Disease

6.5.1 IgA Nephropathy

General Ref

- *Pediatr Nephrol* 2001;16:446
- *Pediatr Nephrol* 2001;16:156
- *N Engl J Med* 2002;347:738

Cause

- Genetic predisposition, associated with HLA BW35, B27, DR1, and DR4

Epidem

- Most common primary glomerulonephritis (GN) disease worldwide; prevalence > in boys; more common in Asians, whites, Native Americans

Pathophys

- Pathogenesis remains unclear. Mesangial IgA deposits histologically.

S+S

- Most common cause of asymptomatic hematuria.
- Associated with respiratory infections, stress, gastroenteritis.
- Gross hematuria usually resolves within days.

Course

- Used to be considered a benign disease; now known 40% progress to chronic renal failure (CRF) in adulthood. Prognosis otherwise good.

Complications

- Hypertension in 10%; CRF

Lab

- Renal biopsy to confirm dx
- No other specific labs
- 50–70% elevated IgA
- Serum IgG, IgM, and C3 usually normal

Rx

- Fish oil (*Semin Nephrol* 2004;24:225), ACEI, steroids

6.5.2 Poststreptococcal Glomerulonephritis

General Ref

- *J Am Soc Nephrol* 2008;19:1855–1864

Cause

- Nephritogenic streptococcus, usually group A streptococcus

Epidem

- Most common immune-mediated nephritis in children, 2M:1F, rare in children < 3 yr; mean age: 7 yr. Incidence in the United States declined significantly over past 2 decades.

Pathophys

- Circulating antigen–antibody complexes deposited in glomerular basement membrane

S+S

- Preceding strep throat or skin infection within 8–14 days, lethargy, anorexia, vomiting, fever, headache, facial edema, flank pain, smoky tea-colored urine, hypertension

Course

- Excellent prognosis; > 90% of children recover completely.
- Microscopic hematuria may persist up to a year.
- Proteinuria resolves within months; if persisting > 6 months, consider alternative dx.

Complications

- Congestive heart failure a rare complication
- Hypertension 50–90%
- Hypertensive encephalopathy 5%

Lab

- Urinalysis: hematuria, proteinuria, RBC casts, granular casts
- Evaluation for strep infection: antistreptolysin-O titer (ASOT), anti-DNase B titers
- Decreased C3 due to activation of alternate complement pathway; returns to normal in 10 d to 8 wk

Rx

- A self-limiting disease; supportive therapy; restrict fluid and salt.
- Oral penicillin V (erythromycin in penicillin allergy) for 10 d.
- Monitoring every 3 months of urine dipstick, urea, electrolytes, and BP to ensure there is no progressive renal failure.

6.5.3 Henoch-Schönlein Purpura Nephritis

General Ref

- *Pediatr Nephrol* 2005;20(9):1269–1272
- *Lancet* 2002;360(9341):1197–1202

Cause

- Immunologically mediated nonthrombocytopenic purpura and systemic vasculitis associated with IgA deposition
- Involves small blood vessels of skin, gi tract, renal tract, and joints

Epidem

- Most common vasculitis in children
- Occurs between 3 and 15 yr; slight male predominance
- 13.5 cases per 100,000 school-aged children per year
- Year-round occurrence but more common in spring, winter, and fall

Pathophys

- Leukoclastic vasculitis with perivascular infiltration of small vessels with polymorphs, mononuclear, and eosinophils
- IgA, C3, and fibrin deposited in walls of affected vessels

S+S

- Often preceding upper respiratory or strep infection. Classic tetrad of involvement:
  - Skin: palpable purpura in pressure-dependent symmetric distribution.

- Joints: arthritis/arthralgia: redness and warmth not common, look for swelling and decreased range of motion.
- Gi tract: abdominal pain, nausea, vomiting, hematochezia. Rarely precede skin rash, typically develop within 1 wk of skin rash (*J Paediatr Child Health* 1998;34(5):405–409).
- Renal disease: microscopic or gross hematuria, isolated proteinuria 2%, nephritic syndrome 2%. Weekly BP and urinalysis for 6 months because a small percentage go on to ESRD.

Course

- Outcome generally excellent if no renal disease
- Better prognosis associated with younger age
- Poorer prognosis in adults
- Resolve within 1 month, 2/3 no further recurrence, 1/3 recurrence with subsequent episodes being milder

Imaging

- Abdominal US (barium enemas will not reduce the intussusception of Henoch Schönlein purpura [HSP] and may damage or perforate the inflamed bowel).
- Doppler flow studies to distinguish orchitis from testicular torsion.

Complications

- Intussusception (edema and hemorrhage of gi tract may act as lead points), orchitis, testicular torsion (*Pediatr Emerg Care* 1992;8:213), priapism, persistent hypertension, protein-losing enteropathy, ESRD

Lab

- No lab test is diagnostic.
- CBC (platelet count is normal), ESR.
- PT, PTT are normal.
- IgA may be elevated in the acute phase.

- Normal or increased IgG and IgM.
- C3 normal (decreased in PSGN and SLE).
- Throat swab for group B strep maybe positive.
- Renal function, urinalysis, stool guaiac.

Rx

- Usually resolves spontaneously.
- Analgesics, NSAIDs for joint pain.
- Avoid aspirin if gi sx.
- Steroids controversial: consider in severe abdominal pain.

6.5.4 Membranoproliferative Glomerulonephritis

General Ref

- *Am J Kidney Dis* 1999;34:1022–1032

Epidem

- Most common 2nd decade of life

Pathophys

- Decreased complement; 3 histologic types I, II, and III

S+S

- Most present with nephritic syndrome with gross hematuria or asymptomatic microscopic hematuria; HT common.

Course

- 50% progress to ESRD 10 yr after first presentation.
- Factors associated with poor prognosis include nephrotic syndrome at presentation, type II, and decreased GFR after 1 yr.

Complications

- HT, ESRD

Lab

- Renal function is normal or decreased.
- Renal biopsy indicated if presenting with nephrotic syndrome in child > 10 yr.
- Significant proteinuria with microscopic hematuria.
- Decrease complement more than 8 wk after presentation with nephritic sx.

Rx

- Treat complications.

6.5.5 Hereditary Glomerulonephritis (Alport's Syndrome)

General Ref

- *Kidney Int* 1993;43:38–44
- *Nephrol Dial Transplant* 2009;24:1464–1471

Cause

- Ref: *Kidney Int* 1993;43(1):38–44
- X-linked 80–85% (mutation in COL4A5 gene on X chromosome)
- Autosomal recessive 15% (genetic defect in COL4A3 or COL4A4 genes)
- Autosomal dominant 5% (heterozygous mutation in COL4A3 and COL4A4 genes)

Epidem

- Most common familial nephritis

Pathophys

- Disorder of basement membrane type IV collagen synthesis
- Alpha IV collagen chains found in basement membrane of kidney, cochlea, and eye

S + S

- Renal: glomerular disease that progresses to ESRD, presenting with asymptomatic microscopic or gross hematuria in the first decade, gradually progressing to proteinuria and hypertension and ESRD in 2nd and 3rd decades.
- Hearing: gradually progressing sensorineural hearing loss, initially for high tones but eventually for all tones.
- Ocular: macular lesions in 20–25%, lenticonus 5%.
- Above classical presentation that occurs in X-linked disease; autosomal recessive similar clinical course with equal severity in males and females; autosomal dominant more gradual loss of renal function.
- Carrier females of X-linked disease are completely normal or may have asymptomatic microscopic hematuria during 3rd–4th decades.

Course

- Progress to ESRD in early adult life

Complications

- ESRD, deafness, leiomyomas found in 2–5% of pts and carriers of X-linked Alport's syndrome

Lab

- Dx confirmed by skin or renal bx, molecular genetic testing

Rx

- No specific treatment; manage complications.
- ACEIs or angiotensin receptor blockers for HT or proteinuria.
- Good BP control may slow progression to ESRD.
- Dialysis or transplant in ESRD.

6.5.6 Glomerulonephritis of Systemic Lupus Erythematosus

General Ref

- World Health Organization Morphologic Classification of Lupus Nephritis (see Table 6.1)

Epidem

- Most common in adolescent girls

Pathophys

- Immune complex deposition in the basement membrane or mesangium

S+S

- Clinical evidence of renal disease in 30–70%; depends on stage

Course

- Aggressive immunotherapy improves prognosis; class IV: high risk of progression to ESRD.

Complications

- ESRD

Lab

- ANA positive.
- Decreased C3 and C4.
- Renal biopsy helps guide immunosuppressive therapy.

Rx

- Should be managed by specialist, including medical and psychosocial support.
- Immunosuppressive therapy: prednisone 1–2 mg/kg per day divided 2 or 3 times daily, then slow taper over 4–6 months once serologic remission has been attained.

Table 6.1 World Health Organization (WHO) Morphological Classification of Lupus Nephritis (modified in 1982)

Class I	Normal glomeruli
	a. Nil (by all techniques)
	b. Normal by light microscopy, but deposits by electron or immunofluorescence microscopy
Class II	Pure mesangial alterations (mesangiopathy)
	a. Mesangial widening and/or mild hypercellularity (+)
	b. Moderate hypercellularity (++)
Class III	Focal segmental glomerulonephritis (associated with mild or moderate mesangial alterations)
	a. With "active" necrotizing lesions
	b. With "active" and sclerosing lesions
	c. With sclerosing lesions
Class IV	Diffuse glomerulonephritis (severe mesangial, endocapillary, or mesangiocapillary proliferation and/or extensive subendothelial deposits)
	a. Without segmental lesions
	b. With "active" necrotizing lesions
	c. With "active" and sclerosing lesions
	d. With sclerosing lesions
Class V	Diffuse membranous glomerulonephritis
	a. Pure membranous glomerulonephritis
	b. Associated with lesions of category II (a or b)
	c. Associated with lesions of category III (a–c)
	d. Associated with lesions of category IV (a–d)
Class VI	Advanced sclerosing glomerulonephritis

Source: Weening JJ, D'Agati VD, Schwartz MM, et al. The classification of glomerulonephritis in systemic lupus erythematosus revisited. *J Am Soc Nephrol.* 2004;15:241–250.

- Class III and IV: 6 months IV cyclophosphamide 500–1000 mg/m^2 then every 3 months for 18 months will decrease renal dysfunction.
- Azathioprine: single dose 1.5–2.0 mg/kg steroid sparing in stages I and II.

6.6 Enuresis

General Ref

- *J Urol* 2006;176:314–324
- *Dev Med Child Neurol* 1989;31:728–736

Terminology

- Primary nocturnal enuresis: nocturnal wetting in a child who has never been dry on consecutive nights for > 6 months
- Secondary nocturnal enuresis: new-onset nighttime wetting on consecutive nights after 6 months or more of dryness
- Incontinence: uncontrollable urine leakage, either continuous or intermittent
- Continual incontinence: constant leakage, ectopic ureter, iatrogenic damage to external sphincter
- Intermittent incontinence: leakage of small amounts day or night: daytime incontinence (old term: *diurnal enuresis*)
- Dysfunctional voiding (now called dysfunctional elimination syndrome): inappropriate muscle contraction during voiding usually associated with constipation

Cause

- Associated with obstructive sleep apnea.
- Diminished bladder capacity.
- Strong evidence of a genetic association: 1 parent, 44% chance; 2 parents, 77% chance; parental age of resolution often predicts child's age of resolution.
- 30% greater incidence in ADHD.
- Thought to be due to neurochemical rather that inattention problem.

Epidem

- Maturational delay: large population study found more fine and gross motor clumsiness, perceptual dysfunction, and speech defects compared with controls.

Pathophys

- Proposed mechanisms include all of the following:
  - Abnormal circadian release of ADH

- Abnormal urodynamics
- Increased atrial natriuretic factor inhibiting renin-angiotensin-aldosterone pathway

S+S

- Nighttime and/or daytime wetting. Physical exam is often unremarkable. Look for bladder distention, fecal impaction, sacral tufts, neuron deficits, labial adhesions, meatal abnormalities.

Course

- Most children eventually become continent in time.

Lab

- Urinalysis, glucose, urine culture and sensitivity

Imaging

- If UTI: US, MCUG

Rx

- Behavioral: alarm therapy 66–70% effective, mechanism likely conditioned response, daily for 3–4 months
- Pharmacologic:
  - Desmopressin first line 0.2 mg (to a maximum of 0.6 mg) 30 min before bed on an empty stomach; synthetic analog of ADH, 60–70% success rate, better if no associated daytime wetting. Use daily for 6 months; then stop for 2 wk and monitor response. Relapse is common.
  - Anticholinergics useful if associated daytime wetting in combination with desmopressin (not so effective alone): Oxybutynin approved in children > 5 yr; tolterodine 2–4 mg off-label use.
  - Imipramine: tricyclic antidepressant; mechanism of action unknown; 64–80% cure rates; only 25% dry on

discontinuing. FDA approved 6–12 yr: 25–50 mg; > 12 yr: 75 mg.

6.7   Proteinuria

General Ref

- *Pediatrics* 2000;105:1242–1249
- *J Pediatr* 1991;119:375–379

Cause

- Transient proteinuria, orthostatic, glomerular disease, tubular disease

Epidem

- Depends on the cause

Pathophys

- Orthostatic: unknown; possible altered renal hemodynamics, partial renal vein obstruction in upright position

S+S

- Common finding on routine urinalysis.
- 10% children 8–15 yr have a positive dipstick at some time.
- Clinical picture will depend on the cause:
  - Renal: fatigue, weight change, facial swelling
  - Transient: recent febrile illness, stress, excessive exercise
- Need to differentiate transient or benign proteinuria from renal disease.
- Transient proteinuria: induced by temperature, exercise, dehydration, stress, resolves spontaneously.
- Orthostatic proteinuria: the most common cause in school-age children, with increased protein excretion in upright position

NEPHROLOGY

and normal excretion in recumbency. Follow up and monitor for renal disease.

- Persistent proteinuria: $> 1+$ proteinuria in multiple 1st morning specimens, over a 3-month period. This requires workup for renal disease (i.e., glomerular or tubular) with possible nephrology referral.

Lab

- Dipstick 1st morning specimen 3 times normal; confirms dx of orthostatic proteinuria.
- Hematuria, casts, and so on, signifies renal origin and needs further workup or referral.

Rx

- Transient benign proteinuria: follow to ensure it resolves; then no evaluation or treatment needed.
- Orthostatic proteinuria: 3 times 1st morning specimen dipsticks, as above. Usually resolves; further workup if not resolving.
- Persistent proteinuria: treat the underlying renal condition.

6.8 Hematuria

General Ref

- *Arch Pediatr Adolesc Med* 2005;159:353–355

Cause

- Glomerulonephritis, clotting disorder, stones, exercise induced, drugs, trauma, benign familial, SS, hemolytic uremic syndrome, HSP, Wilm's tumor, polycystic kidney disease, hypercalcuria

Epidem

- Prevalence 1.5% in pediatrics, mostly transient and intermittent (if associated persistent proteinuria more than $> 1+$, refer to pediatric nephrologist).

S + S

- Depends on the primary cause:
  - Elevated BP, hearing deficit: Alport syndrome
  - Abdominal/flank mass: Wilm's tumor, polycystic kidney disease
  - Rash: HSP, SLE

Course

- Dependent on cause

Lab

- Urinalysis: RBC casts and dysmorphic RBCs diagnostic of a glomerular source.
- Nonglomerular hematuria RBC appearance is similar to those seen in a peripheral blood smear: uniform in size and shape.
- Microscopic hematuria lasting > 1 month warrants further workup.
- Workup will depend on hx and physical and most likely cause: CBC, ASOT, antineutrophil cytoplasmic antibody, renal function, C3 and C4 levels, renal biopsy, hemoglobin electrophoresis, urine calcium.

Imaging

- Every child with gross hematuria should have imaging with abdominal US or CT.

Rx

- Treat the underlying cause.

Chapter 7

Hematology and Oncology

7.1 Anemia

General Ref

- *Pediatr Rev* 1994;15:175–184
- *Pediatr Rev* 2002;23:171–178

Pathophys

- Variety of mechanisms leading to low levels of circulating hgb or rbc volume. Due to blood loss, accelerated rbc breakdown, and slowed rbc production. End consequence can be inadequate oxygen (O_2)-carrying capacity or O_2 delivery. First, r/o iron deficiency.

General Approach

- Look at clinical presentation for direction. Thorough hx: nutritional hx, growth/development, family hx, genetic background, medications, toxic exposures, bleeding.
- Physical exam concentrates on organomegaly, dysmorphic features, limb anomalies.
- Consider full CBC with indexes, smear for morphology, reticulocyte count, specific iron study, haptoglobin, Coombs, hgb electrophoresis.

Iron Deficiency

- Usually dietary cause; typically breastfed infant 6–8 months or child < 2 yr on nonfortified milk. Can be sign of gi blood loss or malabsorption. Exercising teenage girls (menses, gi loss) or use of cow's milk in infants (micro gi losses) exacerbates.
- Lab values: low hgb. Eventually, low mean cell volume (MCV) and high red [blood cell] distribution width (RDW). Reticulocyte count low. Can be severe in rare cases, especially when mixed with other causes of anemia. Platelets often increased.
- Sx: usually asymptomatic; may have recognizable pallor. Toddlers may be irritable, teens fatigued. Complicates plumbism by increasing lead absorption. Can induce hypercoagulable state and more strokes with cyanotic congenital heart disease.
- Iron deficiency occurs prior to anemia; mild anemia often not from iron deficiency. Makes hgb value a poor screen. Low MCV and increased RDW occur with anemia. RDW can help sort from thalassemia minor. Ferritin good screening test but can be artificially elevated with inflammation. Free erythrocyte porphyrin (FEP) also good but affected by lead; iron/total iron-binding capacity (Fe/TIBC) can be affected by chronic disease states. No single test can give certainty to dx.
- Diff dx: if normocytic, low hgb often from viral suppression. In child < 6 months, usually physiologic anemia. If microcytic, various thalassemia traits can mimic. RDW would be normal, and hgb electrophoresis positive (e.g., Southeast Asians have alpha-thalassemia variants not picked up on electrophoresis).
- Prevention: breastfeeding for 6 months or iron-fortified formula. Limit milk intake and/or supplement toddlers with 1 mg/kg iron daily. Supplement teen girls.

- Failure to respond to rx suggests issues with compliance, absorption, ongoing losses, chronic inflammation, or a second hematologic condition: refer.

Ref

- *Pediatr Rev* 2002;23:75–84, 111–122

Beta-Thalassemia

- Genetic defect in hgb synthesis pathway. Homozygotes or blends of different alleles can have severe microcytic anemia with pallor and organomegaly from extramedullary hematopoiesis.
- Homozygotes have mild anemia and low MCV. Often given iron therapy inappropriately.
- Hgb electrophoresis after 6 months of age shows elevated A2 or Fe, and RDW normal. Smear may show basophilic stippling (also seen with lead, not Fe deficiency)
- Alpha-thalassemia (in Southeast Asians) not picked up on usual hgb electrophoresis. Most variants not anemic but low MCV. Rare types can get down to Hgb 7 range. No readily available test and genetics complex.

Hereditary Spherocytosis

- Red cell membrane defect (many variants) leading to increased rbc breakdown. Chronic anemia compensated by increased reticulocyte count, but viral infections (especially parvovirus) can lead to aplastic crises.
- Autosomal dominant; 25% new mutations.
- Can also present with newborn jaundice.
- Lab: anemia, high reticulocyte, and high mean corpuscular hgb concentration. Abnormal osmotic fragility.
- Physical exam: occasionally mild jaundice. Typically splenomegaly. Negative Coombs to r/o immunologic cause. May result in cholelithiasis over time.

- Long-term issue is risks versus benefits of splenectomy. Depends on severity, age.

Transient Erythroblastopenia of Childhood vs Diamond-Blackfan

- Transient erythroblastopenia (TEC) is severe version of "viral suppression"; usually child < 1 yr.
- Main feature is pallor. Need to r/o aplastic anemia (Diamond-Blackfan anemia [DBA]).
- Many with DBA have dysmorphic features, limb anomalies, onset in infancy. More commonly DBA pts have elevated MCV and I antigen, increased rbc adenosine deaminase. Hematology consult indicated to sort all this out.
- TEC may have positive parvovirus titer. Virus has affinity for erythroid marrow precursors.
- TEC shows low hgb and low reticulocyte count. Bone marrow shows lack of rbc precursors. TEC normocytic and normochromic.
- DBA has bad prognosis. Steroid toxicity, iron overload, and evolution to leukemia.
- TEC usually improves over weeks. If hgb < 5, may need transfusion to avoid CHF.

Other Types of Anemia

- Newborn: fetal-placental or fetal-maternal hemorrhage, bleed into cephalohematoma or adrenal, Kasabach-Merritt.
- Physiologic anemia: refers to the normal dip in hgb.

G6PD Deficiency

- Defect in key enzyme of pentose phosphate shunt of glucose pathway; deficiency of NADPH so glutathione reduction inhibited. Oxidative stress from drug/food/illness causes lysis of older cells, with decreased hgb and increased reticulocyte count

- X-linked usually. Usually male (females rare).
- Episodic weakness, jaundice, pallor, fatigue. Neonatal jaundice common and perhaps more susceptible to kernicterus.
- Triggers can include drugs and chemicals (ASA, sulfa, naphthalene, etc.). Mediterranean type set off by fava beans. Most common type in United States is "A-minus" in blacks.

Anemia of Chronic Disease

- Usually mild, rarely down to hgb = 7.
- Inflammatory cytokines inhibit synthetic pathway for incorporating Fe into hgb.
- Lab: MCV normal usually. Fe and TIBC low, ferritin normal (in Fe deficiency, TIBC usually high).
- Rx control of underlying disease. Anemia of renal failure has different mechanism and responds to erythropoietin.

Lead Poisoning

- Leads to anemia only at very high levels (> 60).
- Low or normal MCV. Basophilic stippling.
- Associated anemia usually from concurrent iron deficiency.

Sickle Cell Anemia

- Part of most newborn screening programs.
- Autosomal recessive production of abnormal hgb protein that results in anemia, vaso-occlusion, splenic dysfunction, opsonization defect, increased susceptibility to infection, stroke.
- Pneumococcal prophylaxis indicated for all with use of vaccine, and daily antibiotic prophylaxis in young children, aggressive management of fever.
- Folate given to all.
- Aggressive pain management of "crises" warranted (opiates), in conjunction with hematology consultant.

HEMATOLOGY & ONCOLOGY

- Prophylactic transfusions decrease rates of stroke (*N Engl J Med* 2005;353:2769) but risk of iron overload and other effects.
- Hydroxyurea used in teens with frequent pain episodes.

7.2 Neutropenia

General Ref

- *N Engl J Med* 2000;343:1703

Cause

- Defects of neutrophils
- Congenital neutropenia: recurrent bacterial infections in the 1st yr of life, abscess, cellulitis, meningitis

Rx

- G-CSF

Complications

- Myelodysplastic syndrome (MDS) later in life

Shwachman-Diamond Syndrome

- Presents with exocrine pancreas insufficiency, skeletal abnormalities, recurrent infections of the lung, bone, and skin

Complications

- MDS, leukemia

Rx

- Bone marrow transplant (BMT) is curative.

Cyclic Neutropenia

- Recurrent neutropenia lasting 3–6 d.

- Associated stomatitis, mouth ulcers, and bacterial infections
- Autosomal dominant

Chronic Granulomatous Disease

- *N Engl J Med* 2000;343:1703

Cause

- Mutation causing defect in NADPH oxidase and generation of hydrogen peroxide resulting in defective intracellular killing of pathogens

Epidem

- Two-thirds X-linked; one-third autosomal recessive

Clinical Findings

- Faltering growth, severe bacterial infections: abscess, osteomyelitis in multiple sites in 1st yr of life, pneumonia, lymphadenitis with *Staphylococcus aureus* and *Aspergillus*.

Pathophys

- Impaired neutrophil respiratory burst with nitroblue tetrazolium (NBT). Granuloma formation and an inflammatory process are the hallmark.

Complications

- Pyloric outlet obstruction, bladder outlet obstruction, and rectal fistulae secondary to granuloma formation

Rx

- Prophylactic antibiotics, steroids if granulomas, antifungals and gamma interferon for fungal infections. BMT with matched sibling curative (*Br J Hematol* 2008;140:255).

HEMATOLOGY & ONCOLOGY

Chemotherapeutic Febrile Neutropenia

- Absolute neutrophil count $< 0.5 \times 10^9$ and temperature $> 38°C$ in a pt on chemotherapy.
- This is a medical emergency:
  - Take blood cultures and start on broad-spectrum antibiotics.
  - If fever > 5 d, investigate and treat for a fungal infection, usually with IV amphotericin.
  - Acetaminophen is contraindicated in a child who is not on antibiotics because it may mask fever, but may be given once antibiotics are started.

7.3   Sickle Cell Disease

General Ref

- *Pediatr Rev* 2007;28:259

Cause

- Autosomal recessive inheritance

Epidem

- US blacks 7% trait, 0.5% homozygous.

Pathophys

- A genetic mutation causes a substitution of valine for glutamine on the beta chain of hemoglobin resulting in the formation of HbS, which is unstable at low O_2. Results in formation of sickle cells that stick to vessel walls, causing vascular occlusion resulting in ischemic tissue and organ injury.
- Three main forms:
  - Sickle cell anemia HgbSS: homozygous, all hgb is HbS
  - SC disease HgbSC: cases have HbC (a different point mutation on β-globulin) from one parent and HgbS from the other and no HgbA

- Sickle beta-thalassemia: cases have HgbS from one parent and beta-thalassemia trait from the other; no HgbA, so similar sx to sickle cell anemia.
- Sickle trait: inherit HgbS from one parent and normal hgb from the other. Asymptomatic, but carriers of HgbS so can transmit HgbS to offspring.

S+S

- Presents once fetal hemoglobin levels decrease.
- Fever, pallor, jaundice, splenomegaly, flow murmur.

Clinical Presentations

- Infections: increased susceptibility to encapsulated organisms secondary to hyposplenism; increased incidence of osteomyelitis due to salmonella.
- Painful crisis: acute vaso-occlusive crises precipitated by stress, dehydration, cold, infection, or hypoxia. Any organ can be affected: hand and foot syndrome, dactylitis causing painful swelling of feet and fingers, bone pain, avascular necrosis of femoral head, chest pain with pulmonary infarction, stroke secondary to cerebral infarction.
- Acute anemia: sudden drop in hgb due to:
  - Aplastic crisis: following parvovirus infection, complete but temporary cessation of rbc production.
  - Hemolytic crisis: associated with infection.
  - Sequestration crisis: accumulation of sickled cells in spleen, with abdominal pain, splenic enlargement, and circulatory collapse.
  - Priapism: if not treated urgently with exchange transfusion, may lead to erectile impotence secondary to fibrosis of corpora cavernosa.

Course

- Heterozygous: no clinical disease

- Homozygous: 50% live to 45 yr
- Mortality rate during childhood around 3%, usually from bacterial infections

Complications

- Short stature and delayed puberty, cardiomegaly and heart failure secondary to chronic anemia, pigment gallstones, psychosocial problems

Lab

- CBC, elevated reticulocyte count, PBS (peripheral blood smear) sickled cells
- Chemistry panel: elevated LDH and AST, increased unconjugated bilirubin
- Hb electrophoresis: HbS and increased HbF, dx
- UA, hematuria, low specific gravity, increased reticulocyte count, genetic and antenatal testing available

Xray

- Hair on end skull Xray; step fractures of vertebrae
- Bone scan to differentiate from osteomyelitis
- Chest Xray
- Abdominal US if concerns for cholecystitis
- CT or MRI if concerns re stroke

Rx

- Avoid factors that precipitate vaso-occlusive crises (e.g., cold, stress, dehydration).
- Penicillin prophylaxis from 2 months to 5 yr.
- Pneumococcal vaccination at 2 and 5 yr.
- Folic acid supplements daily, vitamin E 450 iu daily increases rbc survival (*N Engl J Med* 1980;303:454).
- Hydroxyurea: increase HbF, thus diluting HbS and decreasing episodes of painful crises.
- Painful crises:
  - O_2.

- Hydration.
- Oral or IV analgesics.
- May need opiates.
- Antibiotics to treat infection.
- Acute chest syndromes, stroke, and priapism should be treated with exchange transfusion.
- BMT: consider in severe cases with stroke and nonresponse to hydroxyurea. Curative but requires HLA-identical sibling. Cure rate 90%, 5% risk fatal transplant-related complications.

7.4 Neuroblastoma

General Ref

- *J Clin Oncol* 2000;18:3012–3017
- *N Engl J Med* 2002;346:1041–1046
- *J Clin Oncol* 2003;22:4228–4234

Cause

- Embryonal cancer of the peripheral sympathetic nervous system of unknown etiology

Epidem

- Third most common pediatric cancer.
- Accounts for 8% of childhood malignancies.
- 50% of tumors arise from the adrenal gland.
- Median age of dx: 2 yr; 90% diagnosed by 5 yr, and most have disseminated disease at time of dx.

S+S

- Depend on location and can occur anywhere along the sympathetic chain; usually a primary adrenal mass
  - Adrenal: abdominal mass that crosses the midline

- Thoracic: Horner syndrome, airway compression
- Neurologic: myoclonus with opsoclonus: "dancing eyes, dancing feet syndrome," a paraneoplastic syndrome associated with completely chaotic eye movements and cerebellar and truncal ataxia; has a good prognosis
- Skin: raised, tender, bluish nodules
- Bone: bone pain, pancytopenia
- Eyes: heterochromia of the iris, proptosis, raccoon eyes (periorbital bleeding)
- Gi tract: diarrhea, fever, anemia secondary to a VIPoma

Course

- Good prognostic indicators include:
  - Opsoclonus-myoclonus
  - Course < 1 yr
  - Abdominal mass not crossing the midline
  - No amplification of n-myc gene or partial deletion at chromosome 1p

Lab

- CBC and chemistry panel.
- Elevated LDH may have prognostic value.
- Serum ferritin may have prognostic value.
- HVA (homovanillic acid), VMA (vanillylmandelic acid) in 95%; however, false negatives and false positives with these tests so are not useful for screening.
- Pathologic dx at bx.

Xray

- Plain film: calcification at primary site suggestive.
- CT and MRI diagnose a mass or multiple masses.
- Skeletal survey or bone scan to r/o bone lesions.

- Bone marrow bx in all pts for staging.

Rx

- Depend on age at dx and stage of disease:
  - Most are radiosensitive.
  - Chemotherapy for disseminated disease.
  - Low-risk disease: stage 1 or 4S may respond to surgery alone.
  - Advanced disease: stage 4 requires surgery, radiotherapy, and chemotherapy.

7.5 Wilm's Tumor (Nephroblastoma)

General Ref

- *Cancer* 1997;80:2321–2332

Cause

- Familial cases autosomal dominant with variable penetrance; more likely to be bilateral.
- 10–20% associated with tumor-suppressor gene WTI located on chromosome 11p13.
- Associated syndromes: Beckwith-Weidemann syndrome, WAGR (Wilms tumor, aniridia, genitourinary abnormalities, and mental retardation), Denys-Drash syndrome.

Epidem

- Fourth most common childhood tumor
- Most common renal malignancy
- More common in girls than boys
- Annual US incidence 8 case/million children < 15 yr

HEMATOLOGY & ONCOLOGY

S+S

- Most commonly presents with abdominal swelling or painless abdominal mass. There may be some abdominal pain, fever, anorexia, vomiting, hematuria, hypertension, anemia.

Course

- Good prognosis
- More than 90%: 5-yr survival

Lab

- Wbc and differential, electrolytes, serum creatinine and BUN.
- UA, LFTs, serum calcium, coagulation studies.
- Dx based on histology at time of bx or surgical excision.
- Staging based on anatomic extent of tumor.

Imaging

- Abdominal US
- Abdominal CT scan
- Chest Xray

Rx

- Depends on staging and histology.
- If dx suspected, prompt referral to pediatric oncologist and/or surgeon.
- Typical finding of a unilateral tumor: nephrectomy and abdominal lymph node sampling is performed.
- Pts may need postsurgery chemotherapy and radiation if disease more advanced.

7.6 Leukemia

7.6.1 Acute Lymphoblastic Leukemia

General Ref

- *Med Pediatr Oncol* 2002;39:554–557
- *Nat Rev Cancer* 2006;6:193–203

Cause

- 80% of childhood leukemias

Epidem

- Most common cancer of childhood with peak incidence 2–5 yr

Pathophys

- Clonal proliferation of a single lymphoblast that has undergone malignant transformation, with infiltration of leukemic cells into bone marrow, reticuloendothelial system, and other organs, leading to ineffective erythropoiesis

S+S

- Malaise, anorexia.
- Pancytopenia manifests with lethargy, infection, easy bruisability, bone pain.
- Lymphadenopathy, hepatosplenomegaly, superior mediastinal obstruction (uncommon).

Course

- Poor prognostic indicators in acute lymphoblastic leukemia (ALL):
  - Male.
  - Age < 2 yr, > 10 yr.

- Wbc > 50 at dx, high WCC increases the risk of CNS disease.
- Unfavorable cytogenetics: Philadelphia chromosome t(9;22), AML 1 amplification.
- Poor response to induction.
- High levels of residual disease after induction.

Lab

- CBC: increased WCC, neutropenia common, 80% hgb < 10 g/dL, 75% thrombocytopenia
- PBS leukemic lymphoblasts
- Tumor lysis syndrome: increased uric acid, hypocalcium, hyperphosphatemia, hyperkalemia
- Bone marrow aspirate

Imaging

- Chest Xray: mediastinal mass in 5–10% of cases

Rx

- Remission induction 4 wk:
  - Goal: fewer than 5% blasts by 28 d.
  - Before starting treatment, anemia is corrected with blood transfusion, the risk of bleeding minimized by transfusion of platelets, and infection is treated.
  - Additional hydration and allopurinol or urate oxidase are given when the WCC is high to protect renal function against the effects of rapid cell lysis (tumor lysis syndrome).
  - Remission implies eradication of the leukemic blasts and restoration of normal marrow function.
  - 4 wk of combination chemotherapy is given and current induction schedules achieve remission rates of 95%.
- Consolidation:
  - CNS prophylaxis with weekly intrathecal methotrexate
- Maintenance:

- Continue chemotherapy treatment 2 yr for girls and 3 yr for boys.
- Cotrimoxazole is given routinely to prevent *Pneumocystis jiroveci* pneumonia.

7.6.2 Acute Myeloblastic Leukemia

General Ref

- *Cancer* 2005;15(104):788–793

Cause

- 20% of childhood leukemias

Epidem

- Seventh most common pediatric malignancy, M = F, bimodal peak of incidence at 2 yr and 16 yr

Pathophys

- Malignant proliferation of myeloid or nonlymphoid precursors; the proto-oncogene RAS is mutated in up to 30% of acute myeloblastic leukemia (AML).

S+S

- Malaise, anorexia, lethargy, infection, easy bruisability, bone pain, lymphadenopathy, hepatosplenomegaly.
- Less lymph node, intrathoracic and extramedullary disease compared with ALL.
- Systemic involvement is more common than in ALL: proptosis, gum hypertrophy, skin nodules.

Subtypes

- M0 to M5 myeloid differentiating cells
- M6 erythrocyte differentiating cells (erythroblastic leukemia)
- M7 platelet differentiating cells

HEMATOLOGY & ONCOLOGY

Course

- More than 60% survival. Secondary AML from previous chemotherapy has a poorer prognosis.

Lab

- CBC: elevated to low WCC, anemia, thrombocytopenia.
- PBS: myeloblasts.
- Tumor lysis syndrome: increased uric acid, hypocalcemia, hyperkalemia, hyperphosphatemia.
- Bone marrow aspirate: > 30% blasts is dx.
- Immunophenotyping and cytochemistry confirm the dx.

Rx

- General measures: hydration, alkalization, and allopurinol during induction.
- Broad-spectrum antibiotics and antifungals for fever and neutropenia.
- Prophylactic trimethoprim/sulfamethoxazole for *Pneumocystis* infection.
- Four to five courses of intensive myelosuppressive chemotherapy.
- No prolonged maintenance: in high-risk, slow responders, treatment is with allogenic BMT after first remission.

7.7   Hemophilia

General Ref

- *J Pediatr Hematol Oncol* 1998;20:32–35

Cause

- Absence, deficiency, or defective functioning of coagulation factors (F) VIII in hemophilia A or factor IX in hemophilia B

Epidem

- Most common severe inherited coagulation disorder.
- Two-thirds newly diagnosed cases have a family hx; one-third are sporadic.
- Hemophilia A: 80–85% occurring in 1 in 5000 male births.
- Hemophilia B: 10–15% occurring in 1 in 30,000 male births.
- Both are X-linked recessive disorders.
- Hemophilia B more common in Ashkenazi Jews.

Pathophys

- FVIII and FIX are essential for thrombin formation via the intrinsic pathway. In the absence of either factor, generation of thrombin and fibrin is severely impaired.

S + S

- May present in the neonatal period with intracranial hemorrhage (1–2%) or prolonged bleeding from venipuncture, umbilical cord, or circumcision sites.
- In sporadic cases nonaccidental injury may initially be suspected.
- Most children present toward end of 1st yr of life as they start to crawl, walk, and fall.
- Hemarthrosis most often involves the large weightbearing joints: hips, knee, ankles, shoulders, and elbows.
- Graded depending on the level of FVIII or FIX.
- Severe, < 1%: present with spontaneous bleeding into joints and muscles.
- Moderate, 1–5%: bleeding with minor trauma, seldom spontaneous hemorrhage.
- Mild, 5–50%: rare bleeding; only requires factor replacement for surgery.
- Course: depends on degree of deficiency.
- Lab: PT normal, PTT prolonged, von Willebrand factor (vWF) normal, assays of FVIII and FIX reduced.

Rx

- Minor bleeds and simple joint bleeds: treat promptly with IV infusion of recombinant FVIII or FIX to raise circulating levels to 30%.
- Major surgery or life-threatening bleeds: levels need to be raised to 100% then maintained at 30–50% for up to 2 wk to prevent secondary bleeds:
  - FVIII concentrate every 8–12 hr; FIX concentrate every 12–24 hr, with close monitoring of levels.
  - Mild hemophilia A: may be treated with desmopressin (DDAVP). It causes a transient increase in endogenous FVIII and vWF. May be used before surgery for minor procedures and dental extractions (does not work in hemophilia B).
  - Hemophilia B: danazol daily (increases endogenous production).
  - Management should be multidisciplinary, including physical therapists, nursing, psychosocial support.
  - Home treatment is encouraged to decrease the risk of permanent damage. Parents taught replacement therapy from around 2–3 yr, and children can often self-administer by 7–8 yr.
  - Prophylactic treatment to keep FVIII >t 15% is given to children with severe disease to decrease the risk of chronic joint damage.

7.8   Von Willebrand Disease

General Ref

- *J Thromb Haemost* 2006;4:766
- *Blood* 2008;15(111):3998

Cause

- Inherited coagulation disorder due to either quantitative or qualitative disorder of vWF.
- Type 1 is autosomal dominant with variable penetrance.
- Type 2 is autosomal dominant.
- Type 3 is autosomal recessive.

Epidem

- M = F; prevalence in pediatrics 1%.

Pathophys

- vWF facilitates platelet adhesion to damaged endothelium and acts as a carrier protein for FVIII in the peripheral circulation protecting it from inactivation and clearance; thus deficiency results in shorter half-life of FVIII.

S+S

- Easy bruisability, prolonged bleeding after surgery, repeated epistaxis, menorrhagia.
- Type 1: partial deficiency of vWF; most common, accounting for 60–80%; is usually mild; diagnosed at puberty or adulthood.
- Type 2: qualitative deficiency, accounts for 15–20%; tends to have more significant bleeding and is further subdivided into 4 subtypes.
- Type 3: almost complete absence of vWF resulting in secondary deficiency in FVIII accounts for 5% and results in a severe bleeding disorder.

Lab

- PT normal, PTT prolonged, normal bleeding time is prolonged in severe and moderately severe disease and normal in moderate and mild disease
- vWF antigen quantitation.

- Decreased ristocetin cofactor activity (ristocetin causes platelet aggregation in the presence of vWF).
- FVIII normal or decreased.

Rx

- Depends on the type and severity.
- Type 1: local pressure, topical thrombin may be adequate.
- DDAVP for type 1 and 2, ineffective in type 3, stimulates endothelial release of vWF and secretion of FVIII. Use with caution in child < 1 yr due to risk of water retention, resulting hyponatremia, and risk of seizures.

7.9 Lymphoma

7.9.1 Non-Hodgkin Lymphoma

General Ref

- *Blood* 2007;15(109):3479–3488

Cause

- Malignancies of cells of the immune systems; cause is unknown.

Epidem

- Third most common childhood malignancy; M:F: 3:1.

Pathophys

- A firm distinction between solid and hematologic lymphoid malignancy is somewhat artificial because some subtypes of ALL and non-Hodgkin lymphoma (NHL) may represent a continuum of the same disease. In most cases of childhood NHL, the clinical features reflect the pattern of migration of normal lymphoid cells, with lymph nodes the predominant site of disease.

- 30% lymphoblastic: treat as ALL; 90% T cells and 10% B cells.
- 50% mature B cells.
- 20% anaplastic large cell lymphoma.

S+S

- Fever, weight loss, anorexia, fatigue, lymphadenopathy, pain, ascites, abdominal mass, respiratory syndromes/superior vena cava obstruction, bruising, bone pain

Course

- More than 70% survival; relapse associated with very poor prognosis

Lab

- CBC, LFTs, renal function, LDH, and uric acid levels.
- Ascitic, CSF, or pleural fluid for cytology, cytogenics, immunophenotyping.
- Bone marrow aspirate and biopsy may be diagnostic.
- Lymph node bx.

Imaging

- Staging must include radiologic assessment of all nodal sites (CT or MRI) and examination of the bone marrow and CSF.
- Abdominal US
- Chest Xray

Rx

- General measures: pretreatment: hydration, alkalinization, allopurinol to prevent tumor lysis syndrome.
- Lymphoblastic: treat as ALL.
- Intensive multiagent chemotherapy.
- Surgery if total resection can be achieved; avoid extensive surgery.

HEMATOLOGY & ONCOLOGY

7.9.2 Hodgkin Disease

General Ref

- *J Clin Pathol* 2002;55:162–176

Cause

- Unknown

Epidem

- M:F: 2:1
- Bimodal presentation: 15–30 yr and > 50 yr; rare < 5 yr

Pathophys

- Reed-Sternberg cells origin unknown; are the malignant cells of HD.
- Four types:
  - Lymphocyte predominant 10–20%; has the best prognosis
  - Nodular sclerosing 50%; the most common
  - Mixed cellularity 40–50%; most likely to present with extranodal disease
  - Lymphocyte depleted < 10%; rare and worst prognosis

S+S

- Fatigue, anorexia, painless lymphadenopathy.
- Sx include fever, night sweats, and weight loss.

Course

- Depends on the type, with lymphocyte predominant having the best prognosis and lymphocyte depleted the worst.

Lab

- CBC, ESR, LFTs, baseline thyroid function.
- Bone marrow bx, bone scan.

- Lymphangiography (evaluates retroperitoneal adenopathy), optional because it is a technically difficult examination in small children.
- Presence of neoplastic Reed-Sternberg cells in reactive lymph nodes for definitive dx.

Imaging

- Chest Xray for mediastinal masses
- CT chest, abdomen, and pelvis to evaluate for disseminated disease
- CT or MRI of the spine if sx of spinal cord compression

Rx

- Combination chemotherapy, with or without radiotherapy, is the recommended treatment for all stages of the disease. Overall, about 80% of all pts can be cured; for those with disseminated disease, about 60% can be cured.

7.10   Bone Tumors

7.10.1 Ewing Tumor

General Ref

- *N Engl J Med* 1994;4(331):294–299
- *J Clin Oncol* 2001;15(19):1818

Cause

- Derived from red bone marrow. Most lethal malignant bone primary.

Epidem

- M:F: 3:2
- 1% of all childhood cancers and 30% of bone tumors

- Rare in nonwhites
- 2 per 1 million < 20 yr in whites

Pathophys

- 90–95% have translocation associated with cytogenic abnormality, t(11;22) (q24;q12), with fusion genes EWS-FLI1 in this tumor, and 5–10% have the translocation EWS-ERG, t(21;22)(q22;qq12) (*Diagn Mol Pathol* 1998;7:29–35, 1998; *J Pediatr Hematol Oncol* 2001;23:221–224).

S + S

- Affects the flat bones; pain is the earliest symptom; rapidly growing mass. May have fever with differential dx including osteomyelitis and eosinophilic granuloma.

Course

- Poor prognostic factors include:
  - Male sex
  - Older than 12 yr
  - Increased LDH
  - Anemia
  - Poor response to chemotherapy

Lab

- ESR, LDH.
- Alkaline phosphatase: reflects extent of tumor activity.
- Open bx: establishes the dx (needle bx generally does not produce enough material for interpretation).
- Staging with chest Xray, CT chest, MRI of affected bone, bone scan, bone marrow aspiration, and bx.

Rx

- Multidrug therapy (MDT).

- Initial chemotherapy followed by local disease control with surgery or radiotherapy, followed by further chemotherapy.
- Principal chemotherapeutic agents: cyclophosphamide, dactinomycin, doxorubicin, vincristine.
- Newer agents: ifosfamide and etoposide (VP-16).

7.10.2 Osteosarcoma

General Ref

- *Clin Cancer Res* 2005;11:4666
- *Eur J Cancer* 2006;42:2124
- *Cancer* 2009;115:1531

Cause

- Cause unknown
- Increased risk in pts with the germinal mutation for retinoblastoma.
- Increased cancer survival resulting in more cases of radiation-induced osteosarcoma; increased risk associated with alkylating agents.
- Development and progression associated with the recessive oncogenes p53 and RB.

Epidem

- Two times more common than Ewing sarcoma; peaks in teenage yr

S+S

- Affects metaphysis of long bones.
- Most commonly present in distal femur, proximal tibia, and proximal humerus.
- Presents with pain and swelling.
- Adolescents presenting with nonspecific knee pain with no hx of trauma should have Xray.

Course

- Hematogenous spread, 80% lung metastasis, 60–65% survival in nonmetastatic disease

Lab

- Bx

Xray

- Lytic sclerotic or mixed lesions on Xray.
- Advanced disease: characteristic sunburst pattern of periosteal new bone formation.
- Staging with chest Xray and CT chest.
- MRI/angiography for limb salvage operations. Accurately assess intraosseous extension.

Histology

- Differentiates low-grade from high-grade disease

Rx

- Surgery: amputation several centimeters beyond tumor margins.
- High-dose adjuvant chemotherapy has led to increased relapse-free survival.

7.11 Brain Tumors

General Ref

- *Cancer* 2008;15(112):416–432
- *J Clin Oncol* 2007;20(25):1532–1538

Cause

- Almost always primary, 60% infratentorial

Types

- Astrocytoma:
  - 40% of cases and most common.
  - Benign low grade: juvenile cerebellar astrocytoma: slow growing, responds well to surgical treatment.
  - Supratentorial malignant high grade (e.g., glioblastoma multiforme): poor prognosis.
- Medulloblastoma:
  - A primary neuroectodermal tumor accounting for 20% of cases.
  - Nearly always arise in midline of posterior fossa/ cerebellum.
  - Presents with headache, vomiting, and ataxia.
  - Most common high-grade tumor.
  - Commonly metastasis within and is the only type that can metastasize outside the CNS.
  - Prognosis: 50% 5-yr survival with CNS irradiation following surgical resection.
- Ependymoma:
  - 8% of cases
  - Behaves like a medulloblastoma mostly arising from the posterior fossa but can also arise from ventricles and spinal cord.
- Brain stem glioma:
  - 6% of cases peak in early childhood.
  - Presents with cranial nerve defects, ataxia, and pyramidal tract signs.
  - Bx is dangerous, so diagnosed with CT or MRI.
  - Prognosis: < 20% survival.
  - Rx: radiotherapy palliative; no place for chemotherapy.
- Craniopharyngioma:
  - 8% of cases
  - Developmental tumor arising from remnants of Rathke pouch.

- Locally invasive, presenting with raised intracranial pressure, visual field defects, pituitary dysfunction.

Epidem

- Most common solid tumor in childhood. Almost always primary, 60% infratentorial.

Pathophys

- S+S: headache (classically worse on lying down)
- Vomiting (especially on waking in the mornings)
- Papilledema
- Squint secondary to VI nerve palsy
- Nystagmus
- Ataxia
- Personality or behavior change

Course

- The functional implications of the site of the tumor, the potential hazards of surgery, and the importance of radiotherapy in treatment all combine to place children with brain tumor at particular risk of neurologic disability and of growth, endocrine, and neuropsychological problems.

Lab

- MRI and CT head.
- LP should be avoided if any signs of raised intracranial pressure.

Rx

- Strongly influenced by the anatomic position of the tumor

Chapter 8
Neurology

8.1 Duchenne Muscular Dystrophy

General Ref

- *NY Acad Sci* 2009;1175:71–79
- *Lancet* 2002;359:687–695

Cause

- Duchenne muscular dystrophy (DMD) is a severe muscle-wasting disease caused by frame shifting and nonsense mutations in the dystrophin gene.

Epidem

- Most common muscular dystrophy, incidence 1 in 3500, onset 3–5 yr of age

Pathophys

- Mutation of dystrophin gene on chromosome Xp21, which maintains the integrity of the muscle wall.
- Deficiency of dystrophin production results in influx of calcium ions, a breakdown of the calcium calmodulin complex, and an excess of free radicals. This leads to irreversible destruction of muscle cells and severe progressive muscle weakness.

S+S

- Proximal myopathy, frequent falls, waddling gait, lumbar lordosis, selective atrophy of muscles leading to calf pseudo-hypertrophy, cardiomyopathy: resting tachycardia may be an early sign; Gower sign.

Course

- Characterized by progressive muscle deterioration that results in pts becoming wheelchair-dependent around 13 yr of age, with death from respiratory failure and cardiomyopathy in their 20s.

Complications

- Contractures, osteoporosis, and increased fracture risk
- Scoliosis, lordosis
- Rapid shallow breathing pattern due to decreased vital capacity

Lab

- EKG tall R waves and deep Q waves
- Echocardiogram
- Creatinine kinase 50–100 times normal
- Increased transaminases; increased LDH
- Molecular DNA studies: PCR and Southern blot assay
- EMG and NCS now less widely used due to availability of molecular genetics

Rx

- Supportive:
  - Good nutrition to avoid obesity; daily calcium and vitamin D.
  - Exercise as tolerated.
  - Psychosocial support.

- Physical therapy, passive stretching, nighttime splinting, good posture.
- Prednisone started at 6–12 yr can prolong walking for 1–2 yr; mechanism for this is effect is unknown; deflazacort has shown similar benefits.
- No effective treatment is currently available.
- Clinical trials: development of antisense-mediated exon skipping as a treatment for DMD, spinal muscular atrophy (SMA), and myotonic dystrophy (*Curr Opin Neurol.* 2009;22(5):532–538).

8.2   Cerebral Palsy

General Ref

- *Cochrane Database Syst Rev* 2007;(2):CD004149
- *Gastrointest Endosc* 1999;50:183–188

Cause

- Damage or dysfunction of the brain resulting in nonprogressive motor impairment

Subtypes

- Spastic: 40%; increased deep tendon reflexes, clonus, hypertonia
- Spastic diplegia: lower extremity involvement
- Spastic hemiplegia: one side of the body
- Spastic quadriplegia: total body involvement
- Dyskinetic: 30%; total body involvement with fluctuating tone and rigidity
- Athetoid: slow writhing movement
- Dystonic: posturing of head trunk and extremities
- Ataxia: 10%; characteristic cerebellar signs
- Mixed: 10%; 2 or more types with spastic and dyskinetic most common

NEUROLOGY

- Other: 10%; criteria for CP met but subtype cannot be defined

Epidem

- 50% associated with prematurity.
- Increased concordance with monozygotic vs dizygotic twins.
- IUGR more common in CP.
- Hypoxic ischemic encephalopathy accounts for 9% cases of CP.

Pathophys

- Chorioamnionitis associated with CP, premature babies vulnerability of periventricular white matter at 28–32 wk results in periventricular leukomalacia associated with IUGR.

S+S

- Prenatal: exposure to toxins, infections, vaginal bleeding, preeclampsia, breech, preterm labor, IUGR, placental disorders
- Perinatal: neonatal resuscitation, low APGARs, birth trauma, evidence of neonatal encephalopathy
- Postnatal: infection, trauma, metabolic, severe delay in milestones

Lab

- Hearing and vision assessment, genetic and metabolic labs depending on hx

Xray

- Brain imaging if hydrocephalus suspected

Rx

- Family-centered care to optimize function and decrease handicap

Interdisciplinary

- Education services: recent emphasis on inclusion and mainstreaming.
- Physical therapy/occupational therapy/strength training.
- Early referral to pediatric orthopedics.
- Early referral for developmental assessment.
- Some studies suggest benefits of injections of botulism toxin A in children with increased muscle tone affecting function (*Dev Med Child Neurol* 1994;36:386–396; *Int J Clin Pract* 2002;56:564–567).
- Constraint-induced movement therapy used more in hemiplegic CP: Goal of therapy is to increase use of affected limbs (*Cochrane Database Syst Rev* 2007;(2):CD004149).

8.3   Headaches

General Ref

- *Neurology* 2002;59:490
- *Neurology* 2004;63:427

Cause

- Primary: migraine, tension, cluster headache, trigeminal autonomic cephalgias
- Secondary: due to another underlying cause (e.g., HT, CNS infection, sinusitis, dental pain)

Epidem

- M:F: 1:2
- Prevalence: 57–82% by 15 yr
- Boys: stable prevalence 7–14 yr; decline thereafter
- Girls: increased prevalence 7–22 yr

Pathophys

- Complex interplay of genetics, emotion, environment, and hormonal factors.
- Vasodilation and perivascular inflammation influenced by hormones and circadian rhythms, bioactive amines, substance P, and serotonin.
- Migraine headaches (*Pediatr Rev* 2007;28:43):
  - Interictal neuronal hyperexcitability with cortical spreading depression is the basis for aura.
  - Headache due to trigeminal nerve activation at peripheral and central level.

Sx

- Good hx helps delineate cause, nocturnal vs diurnal, wakes pt up, intensity, personality changes, ataxia, visual weakness, precipitants such as anxiety, school, stress, past medical hx, drugs and alcohol use

Symptoms

- Abnormal BP, neuro-cutaneous stigmata, signs of trauma, nuchal rigidity, signs of raised intracranial pressure on fundoscopic exam
- Red flags: dramatic increase in severity, wakes child from sleep, change in headache pattern, first or worst headache

Lab

- Not usually necessary for primary headache

Xray

- Imaging unnecessary in the absence of sx and si of raised intracranial pressure or abnormal neurologic signs

Rx

- Psychological support.

- Identify and avoid triggers.
- NSAIDs or acetaminophen.
- Antiemetics.
- Serotonin agonists.
- Treat the cause in secondary headaches.

8.4 Childhood Periodic Syndromes

8.4.1 Cyclic Vomiting Syndrome

General Ref

- *J Pediatr Gastroenterol Nutr* 2008;47:379–393
- *J Pediatr Gastroenterol Nutr* 1993;17:361–369

Cause

- Unknown

Epidem

- 2.5% schoolchildren, 9.6 yr average age of dx; M = F

Pathophys

- Unknown
- Associated with migraine
- Linked with food allergies (*Eur J Pediatr* 2000;159:360–363), endocrine, metabolic, mitochondrial disorders
- Associated with cessation of chronic cannabis use

S+S

- Three essential features:
  - Stereotypical pattern of acute episode of vomiting at least 4 times per hr with no signs of gi disease.
  - Three or more episodes per yr.
  - Absence of nausea and vomiting between episodes.

- Attacks last 1 hr to 5 d; 50% children have attacks at regular intervals every 2–4 wk; the rest unpredictable temporal pattern. Two-thirds of parents can identify a trigger, usually infectious (upper respiratory tract infection) or psychological.
- Supporting evidence: family hx of migraine, self-limiting nature.
- Nausea and lethargy are key features.
- Associated sx: nausea, headache, abdominal pain, motion sickness, photophobia.

Course

- Many children outgrow CVS by preteen to early teen yr; up to 75% go on to develop migraine by 18 yr

Lab

- CBC, comprehensive metabolic panel (CMP), UA; metabolic screen to r/o other cause

Xray

- Consider upper gi series/small bowel follow-through, CT or MRI of head if dx not clear from hx

Rx

- Supportive during episodes.
- If severe, admission for IV fluids, antiemetics.
- Look for and avoid triggers (motion sickness: car rides; food allergy: chocolate, cheese).
- Migraine prophylaxis can be effective if family hx of migraine.
- Goal: abort and shorten episode; anecdotal evidence of improvement with Zofran and sedation (diphenhydramine and lorazepam).

8.4.2 Abdominal Migraine

General Ref

- *Pediatrics* 2005;115:812–815

Cause

- Unknown

Epidem

- Affects up to 12% of school-age children

Pathophys

- Unknown

S+S

- Recurrent attacks of midline, periumbilical, poorly localized, dull moderate to severe abdominal pain lasting 1–72 hr.
- Two or more other features: anorexia, nausea, vomiting, pallor.
- No headache and physical exam exclude other causes.

Complications

- Many children evolve to migraine.

Lab

- To exclude other causes

Xray

- To exclude other causes

Rx

- Migraine treatment may be effective.

8.5   Benign Paroxysmal Vertigo

General Ref

- *Brain Dev* 2001;23:38–41

Cause

- Unknown; often family hx of migraine

Epidem

- Most frequent cause of vertigo in children; often presents in toddler although may manifest later in childhood

Pathophys

- Unknown

S+S

- Recurrent attacks of severe vertigo resolving spontaneously in minutes to hr.
- Child may appear frightened and off-balance during episodes.
- No loss of consciousness; may be nausea, vomiting, sweating, and nystagmus.
- Vestibular and audiometric exams all normal between attacks.

Course

- Resolves spontaneously and evolves into migraine

Xray

- EEG normal

Rx

- Usually resolves spontaneously. Main aim is to r/o epilepsy.

8.6   Benign Paroxysmal Torticollis

General Ref

- *Clin Pediatr (Phila)* 1984;23:272–274
- *Brain Dev* 2000;22:169–172

Cause

- Unknown; often family hx of migraine

Epidem

- Occurs in younger children

Pathophys

- Unknown; considered to be a migraine equivalent

S+S

- Attacks of head tilt, vomiting, and ataxia lasting from hr to d. Episodes less frequent with age and have usually resolved by 5 yr.

Course

- Self-limited condition

Xray

- EEG.
- MRI to r/o posterior fossa disease will be normal.

Rx

- No specific medications have been found to be effective in preventing recurrence.

8.7   Guillain-Barré Syndrome

General Ref

- *Neurology* 2003;61:736
- *Arch Dis Child Educ Pract Ed* 2007;92:161

Cause

- Preceding infectious disease in 50–67%; viral or bacterial infection, surgery, immunization, lymphoma, or exposure to toxins

Epidem

- 0.5 to 1.5/100,000 < 18 yr.
- Most common cause of acute flaccid paralysis in countries with modern vaccination program.
- Bimodal distribution peaks in young adults 15–35 yr and elderly 50–75 yr.

Pathophys

- An acute inflammatory autoimmune neuritis caused by T-cell response to peripheral myelin. Demyelination occurs in peripheral nerves and nerve roots.

S+S

- Criteria for dx: areflexia, rapidly progressive symmetric weakness of 2 or more limbs, course less than 4 wk, other disorders excluded.
- Supportive criteria: sensory sx rare: occasional pain, cranial nerve involvement, absence of fever (if present consider an alternative dx), typical CSF findings, preceding febrile illness.
- Classic Guillain-Barré syndrome (GBS): acute flaccid paralysis, pain, paresthesia, areflexia, cranial neuropathies.

- Miller Fisher: GBS variant: acute onset of triad of areflexia, ataxia, and ophthalmoplegia preceding *Campylobacter jejuni* infection common.

Course

- In mild cases, axonal function remains intact and recovery can be rapid if remyelination occurs.
- In severe cases, axonal degeneration occurs, and recovery depends on axonal regeneration. Recovery becomes much slower, and there is a greater degree of residual damage.
- Recent studies on the disorder have demonstrated that approximately 80% of the pts have myelin loss, whereas in the remaining 20% the pathologic hallmark of the disorder is indeed axon loss.

Lab

- LP: CSF has elevated protein level (100–1000 mg/dL), without an accompanying pleocytosis (increased cell count). A sustained pleocytosis may indicate an alternative dx, such as infection.
- Electrodiagnosis: EMG may show prolonged distal latencies, conduction slowing, conduction block, and temporal dispersion of compound action potential in demyelinating cases. In primary axonal damage, the findings include reduced amplitude of the action potentials without conduction slowing.

Xray

- MRI of the spine in a child presenting with paraparesis. MRI findings of spinal nerve root enhancement support dx of GBS.

Rx

- Immediate admission if slightest suspicion of GBS, with ICU admission at first sign of compromise.

NEUROLOGY

- Respiratory monitoring with serial vital capacity and intubate if any concern of impending compromise.
- Autonomic monitoring.
- Careful fluid balance.
- Avoid complications of pressure phenomena: compressive neuropathies, bed sores.
- Childhood GBS motor disability grading scale:
    0   Healthy
    1   Minor si and sx
    2   Able to walk 5 m without support
    3   Able to walk 5 m but need support
    4   Bed- or chair-bound; unable to walk 5 m
    5   Requires ventilatory assistance
    6   Dead
- Specific rx: immunomodulatory, IVIG, plasmapheresis, no steroids

8.8   Seizures

General Ref

- *Pediatr Rev* 2007;28(10)

Diff Dx

- Confirm seizure: differential includes breath holding, apnea, syncope, anxiety/hyperventilation, vertigo, migraine, psychiatric (acute confusional state, psychogenic seizures, explosive behavior, ADHD), parasomnia (sleepwalking, night terror), narcolepsy, cataplexy, tics, dystonia, masturbation, GE reflux (Sandifer), dysrhythmia (cardiac), stroke, hyperexplexia.
- Once confirmed, identify type: idiopathic or symptomatic epilepsy. Underlying causes: brain malformations, tumors,

trauma, infection, stroke, arteriovenous malformation, metabolic disorders or derangements (glucose, calcium, pyridoxine), hypoxic injury, toxins, medication reactions, inborn errors.

- Classification system:
  - Generalized vs partial:
    - Generalized includes tonic-clonic (classic grand mal), tonic, clonic, myoclonic, absence (classic petit mal), or atonic. Always begin with loss of consciousness because bilateral discharges at onset.
    - Partial seizures can be with retained consciousness (simple partial) or impaired (complex partial) or focus can spread and become generalized (secondary generalized tonic-clonic).
  - Seizure syndromes in childhood:
    - Lennox-Gastaut syndrome: onset age 3–5 yr of mixed seizure types: absence, tonic-clonic, atonic, myoclonic. EEG shows slow spikes. Usually associated with severe developmental delays. Difficult to treat: valproate, with multiple other drugs as adjuncts often needed. Ketogenic diet helpful. Vagal nerve stimulator may help.
    - Rolandic epilepsy (benign partial epilepsy with centrotemporal spikes): onset 3–13 yr. Seizures often nocturnal. Can begin with facial foci: drooling or paresthesias. Often familial (autosomal dominant). Carbamazepine first line if rx needed. Outgrown by adulthood. Recommend imaging to r/o parasagittal lesion.
    - Juvenile myoclonic epilepsy: presents in teens (12–18 yr). Often familial (dominant). Characteristic EEG with fast spike and wave. Have myoclonic jerks when awakening, with or without associated absence or tonic-clonic events. Valproate traditional first-line rx, but lamotrigine and others show promise. Typically need lifelong treatment.

- Infantile spasms (West syndrome): begin at 4–18 months with sudden brief symmetric axial muscle contractions. Often come in clusters as awakening or going to sleep; can be set off by loud noises. Usually less responsive after spasms. Associated with tuberous sclerosis. Typical hypsarrhythmia on EEG. Vigabatrin is drug of choice although not approved. GABA inhibitor. Infants usually end up with MR. Spasms outgrown by 3–4 yr, but 60% have other seizure types.
- Typical absence seizures: school aged, presenting with brief abrupt losses of awareness. Often with eyelid fluttering. Typical EEG pattern with 3-cps symmetric spike and waves. No postictal phenomena; usually developmentally normal. Outgrown by adolescence or young adulthood. Ethosuximide usually first-line rx.
- Refining the dx:
  - H+P are key, with ancillary tests supplementing. Consider details of event, including possible infectious or toxic triggers. EEG typically done; neuroimaging when focal quality or associated developmental abnormalities. MRI is gold standard. EEG can be normal with true seizures but rarely normal if daily new-onset spells.

Rx

- Consult pediatric neurologist for rx depending on seizure type.

8.9 Port Wine Stains

General Ref

- *Pediatr Clin North Am* 2000;47(4):783–812
- *Pediatrics* 1999;87(3):323–327
- *Ann Plast Surg* 2006;57(3):260–263

Cause

- Congenital vascular malformations that do not involute spontaneously; composed of mature dermal capillaries

Epidem

- Occurs in 0.5% of newborns, most commonly affecting the face.
- Associated with certain syndromes:
  - Sturge-Weber syndrome: triad of facial port wine stain (PWS), glaucoma, and leptomeningeal angiomatosis; 6–8% have facial PWS involving ophthalmic division of trigeminal nerve.
  - Klippel-Trenaunay syndrome: PWS, bone and soft tissue extremity hypertrophy, venous varicosity usually on the leg
  - Cobb syndrome: PWS in dermatomal distribution

Pathophys

- Vascular malformation of mature dilated dermal capillaries

S+S

- Present at birth.
- Pink to purple macules.
- Usually unilateral, most commonly affecting the head and neck.
- If associated with syndromes, si and sx are those of the syndrome (e.g., MR and seizures in Sturge-Weber, limb hypertrophy in Klippel-Trenaunay).

Course

- Do not involute spontaneously

Rx

- Pulsed dye laser therapy avoids thermal injury to surrounding tissues and improvement occurs without scarring.

8.10   Acute Disseminated Encephalomyelitis

General Ref

- *Neurology* 2007;68:S7
- *Arch Neurol* 2005;62:1673
- *Pediatr Infect Dis J* 2004;23:756

Cause

- Etiology unknown

Epidem

- M = F, with average age of onset 5–8 yr
- More common in children (*Neurol Clin* 2003;21:745)

Pathophys

- Acute or subacute inflammatory demyelinating event affecting multiple areas in the CNS with polysymptomatic presentation
- Encephalopathy with behavioral changes and alterations in consciousness invariable
- By definition no prior episodes and no alternative etiologies

S+S

- Preceding viral illness or vaccination.
- Nonspecific neurologic sx suggesting area involved.
- Typically complete recovery from routine illness with an interval of wellness followed by mental status changes.
- Mental status changes are required to make the dx.

Complications

- Adverse cognitive outcomes: behavioral problems, cognitive impairment (*Pediatr Neurol* 2003;29:117; *Pediatr Neurol* 2004;31:191).

Lab

- LP: increased protein, occasional oligoclonal bands
- EEG slow wave abnormalities, nonspecific signs of an encephalopathic process

Imaging

- Head CT: 40% sensitivity (normal CT does not r/o dx).
- MRI: Predominant white matter lesions with large, bilateral, asymmetric multifocal lesions.

Rx

- High-dose steroids: IV methylprednisolone 10–30 mg/kg per d for 3–5 d. Then oral steroid taper for 4–6 wk.
- Plasmapheresis may be successful if above fails.

8.11   Restless Legs Syndrome

General Ref

- *Sleep Med* 2003;4:101–119
- *Mayo Clin Proc* 2004;79:916–922

Cause

- Familial cases suggest a genetic component (*Ann Intern Med* 1995;122:174).
- Primary form idiopathic with cause unknown.
- Secondary form associated with diabetes mellitus, iron deficiency anemia, ESRD, MS.

Epidem

- Prevalence: children 8–17 yr 2%; if parent affected, prevalence increases to 70%.

S+S

- The International Restless Legs Study Group have proposed 4 criteria for dx:
  - An urge to move the legs, usually accompanied or caused by uncomfortable and unpleasant sensations in the legs.
  - The urge to move or unpleasant sensations begin or worsen during periods of rest or inactivity such as lying or sitting.
  - The urge to move or unpleasant sensations are partially or totally relieved by movement, such as walking or stretching, at least as long as the activity continues.
  - The urge to move or unpleasant sensations are worse in the evening or only occur in the evening. When sx are severe, the worsening at night may not be noticeable but must have been previously present.
- Supportive criteria for the dx of restless legs syndrome (RLS) include the following:
  - A family hx of RLS
  - A positive response to dopaminergic drugs
  - Periodic limb movements during wakefulness or sleep as assessed with polysomnography or leg activity devices

Lab

- CBC, ferritin level

Rx

- An expert panel has devised a treatment algorithm based on dividing RSL into three types: intermittent, daily, and refractory (*Mayo Clin Proc* 2004;79(7):916–922).
  - Intermittent RLS: sx infrequent but bothersome enough to require treatment but not daily medication. Treatment options include:
    - Nonpharmacologic therapy: avoiding triggers: caffeine, nicotine, and alcohol; iron replacement; mental agility

exercises. Levodopa, dopamine agonists, low-potency opioids or opioid agonists, benzodiazepines or benzodiazepine agonists.

- Daily RLS: frequent sx requiring daily treatment. Treatment options include:
  - Nonpharmacologic therapy as above, dopamine agonists, gabapentin, low-potency opioids or opioid agonists
- Refractory RLS: daily sx treated with a dopamine agonist but with a poor response. Referral to a specialist for RLS management should be considered for these pts. Four different pharmacologic treatment approaches are recommended: change to gabapentin; change to a different dopamine agonist; add a second agent such as gabapentin, a benzodiazepine, or an opioid; or change to a high-potency opioid or tramadol.

NEUROLOGY

Chapter 9

Endocrinology

9.1　Precocious Puberty

General Ref

- *Pediatrics* 2002;109:E30
- *J Pediatr* 2006;149:532–536

Cause

- Defined as signs of puberty in a girl < 8 yr of age and in a boy < 9 yr of age.
- Associated factors:
  - Environmental factors (e.g., obesity and estrogen-containing substances such as tea tree oil, lavender oil associated with reports of gynecomastia in males)
  - Psychosocial factors: adopted children moving from under-nourished to well-nourished situation associated with early puberty

Epidem

- Higher incidence in girls

S+S

- Estrogen effect: breast development, vaginal secretions, and menses

- Androgen effect: pubic hair, axillary hair, and growth of the genitalia in a male or clitoromegaly in a female
- Normal puberty:
  - In girls:
    - Breast buds begin around 10 yr of age
    - Followed by pubic hair 6 months later
    - First period 12 yr, 9 months of age in whites and 9 months earlier in African Americans
  - In boys:
    - Testicular enlargement begins around 11 yr, 6 months of age
    - Followed by pubic hair
    - Followed by maturation around the age of 15 yr
- Normal variants:
  - Benign premature thelarche: unilateral or bilateral, begins 6 months to 2–3 yr.
  - No growth spurt, no vaginal bleeding, no pubic hair; ultimately regresses and true puberty occurs at the normal time.
  - Benign premature adrenarche: activation of the adrenal glands resulting in underarm hair, pubic hair, body odor or acne, all manifestations of adrenal hormones and can occur in boys or girls between 3–8 yr, no clitoromegaly, no breast development, and no growth spurt. More common in African Americans and obese children. Remainder of puberty typically happens at the normal time.
- Pathologic early puberty:
  - Central precocious puberty (CPP)/gonadotropin dependent:
    - Early production of LH and FSH from the pituitary, so may get breast and pubic hair development and usually associated with a significant growth spurt. If the child is not treated, will be significantly shorter as adult.

- More common in girls and much more likely to be benign.
- < 10% girls presenting with CPP have any pathologic findings.
- Less common in boys, but up to 50% of boys have an abnormal lesion, usually in the CNS.
- All boys and any girl presenting < 7 yr of age should have imaging of the brain.
- Gonadotropin-independent precocious puberty:
  - LH and FSH are suppressed (not in the pubertal range, as found in CPP).
  - Causes include autonomously functioning ovarian, testicular, or adrenal lesions.
  - Exogenous causes: important to screen for because more common; exposure to estrogen or androgen creams in the household (e.g., mother using AndroGel cream for arthritis, Premarin cream on face for wrinkles).

Lab

- Signs of adrenarche only; evaluation includes sex steroids from the adrenal glands, US to look at adrenals, bone age.
- Signs of thelarche only; evaluation includes estradiol, LH, FSH, bone age.
- If estrogen is high but LH and FSH are suppressed, do an US to look at the adrenals and ovaries.
- If LH and FSH are high, do an MRI head scan to look for cause of CPP.
  - NB: Must do highly sensitive assay for LH and FSH in children; standard tests are designed to pick up higher levels in women.
  - Do not do bone age < 2 yr because there are not enough epiphyses to get a good bone age; > 2 yr will give an idea of skeletal maturation.

Rx

- Goals:
  - To prevent short stature, which is a concern in early presentation (not a concern if presenting > 7.5 yr of age).
  - Prevent menses in a young girl, which can be psychosocially difficult to accept.
  - Prevent sexual abuse.
  - Electing not to treat is reasonable, especially if only slightly early.
- Depo Lupron: can be given once monthly or once every 3 months:
  - Doesn't stop adrenarche but prevents progression of breast development and menses.
  - Fewer than 5% have an allergic reaction causing a sterile abscess.
  - May bleed after first injection, but no periods thereafter.
  - Quickly reversible.
  - Normal fertility, normal bone density in women treated as children.
  - Limiting factor is cost: $9600 per yr.
- Alternative: PO Provera daily or twice daily tablet:
  - Only effect is to stop the period
  - Does not prevent development of breasts
  - Does not do anything to preserve height
  - Does not affect adrenarche
- Time to stop whichever treatment modality is used is in the 11th yr

9.2   Pubertal Delay

General Ref

- *J Clin Endocrinol Metab* 2002;87:1613–1620
- *J Pediatr* 1995;126:545–550

Def

- No testicular enlargement by 14 yr in boys; no breast development by 13 yr in girls *or* breast development starts but 5 yr later period has not started.

Cause

- Normal variant most common.
- Central process: LH and FSH fail to increase due to abnormality at the pituitary or hypothalamic levels.
- Primary problem with testis or ovaries.

Epidem

- 90–95% constitutional delay and, of these, 60% have a positive family hx.

S+S

- Constitutional delay:
  - Most common cause.
  - Unremarkable past medical hx, normal birth weight, then ≤ 5th percentile by first 2 yr of life but following a normal growth curve.
  - Usually late to have teeth erupt.
  - Otherwise healthy; no chronic illnesses.
  - Often a family hx of late bloomers.
  - Physical exam shows no signs of thelarche or adrenarche.
- Gonadal failure:
  - Turner syndrome: streak ovaries, ovarian failure
  - Klinefelter syndrome: do go into puberty but have small testes
  - Cancer survivors: gonads damaged by radiation or chemotherapy

- Central hypogonadism:
  - Anorexia nervosa and amenorrheic athletes (if starts 9th to 10th yr will affect final height but if begins at 15 yr, final height unaffected but bone health affected)
  - Children on high-dose steroids that suppress the hypothalamic-pituitary-gonadal axis
  - CNS tumors

Lab

- Look for chronic disease.
- TSH.
- Bone age.
- GH if short stature.
- Karyotype for Turner or Klinefelter syndromes.
- Low estrogen and testosterone in all these conditions, including constitutional delay.
- Low LH, FSH, and delay in pubic hair development in constitutional delay.
- Gonadal failure: LH and FSH are high and pubic hair may be present.
- Central LH and FSH are low; normal pubic hair.

Rx

- Constitutionally delayed male: reassurance or give short priming dose of testosterone 100 mg monthly for 3 months; immediate physical changes, growth of penis, pubic hair that psychologically can really make a difference.
- Other causes: start low and slowly increase doses of sex steroids in consultation with an endocrinologist.

9.3   Short Stature

General Ref

- *J Clin Endocrinol Metab* 2008
- *J Clin Endocrinol Metab* 2002;87:1402–1406

Def

- Height < 3rd percentile or height crossing percentile charts downward. Most normal, but the more pronounced the short stature, the more likely there will be a pathologic cause.

Causes

- Familial: defined as height < 3rd percentile with skeletal age appropriate for chronologic age and normal growth rate. Most short children have short parents and child falls within mid-parental height percentile target range. Consider that both parents and child could be suffering from a pathologic cause.
- Constitutional delay of growth and puberty: delayed puberty that is often familial. More common in boys and is a variation of normal. Associated with excessive dieting and physical training. If problems with bullying, poor self-esteem, then puberty may be induced with androgens and estrogens.
- IUGR: about 1/3 of children born with severe IUGR or who are very premature remain short.
- Chromosomal disorders: Prader-Willi syndrome, Down syndrome. Usually diagnosed at birth but Russell Silver, Turner, Noonan may present with short stature. All short girls with subnormal growth rates should have banded karyotyping for Turner syndrome as part of their workup.
- Skeletal disorders: skeletal dysplasias resulting in poor growth may not be obvious. They present with disproportionate short

stature that can be confirmed by measuring: sitting height (base of spine to top of head) and subischial leg length (subtraction of sitting height from total height) and plotting on charts that assess normality of body proportions. Radiologic studies can also be helpful.

- Nutritional disorders: an important worldwide cause of short stature. This may be due to insufficient food (protein energy malnutrition in developing countries), restricted diets (anorexia nervosa an important cause in the United States), poor appetite from chronic illness (e.g., celiac disease, inflammatory bowel disease, CF).
- Psychosocial deprivation: physical and emotional deprivation is associated with short stature, poor weight gain, and delayed puberty. These children show catch-up growth and may have precocious puberty if placed in a nurturing environment.
- Endocrine disorders:
  - Congenital hypothyroidism is diagnosed soon after birth so not associated with abnormal growth. In childhood, hypothyroidism is usually caused by autoimmune thyroiditis and is characterized by subnormal linear growth rate, delayed bone age, and increased weight.
  - GH deficiency may be an isolated defect. Presents with subnormal growth rate and markedly delayed bone age. It may also be secondary and associated with other pituitary deficiencies as in the following: septo-optic dysplasia, head injuries, CNS infections, cranial irradiation.
- Craniopharyngioma is the most common tumor associated with panhypopituitarism and usually presents in childhood with headache, visual disturbances (optic atrophy, bitemporal hemianopsia), neurologic sx, and sometimes growth failure.
- Major organ system disease: any chronic illness—CNS, cardiac, pulmonary, renal, gi, or hematologic disorders—can present with poor linear growth and short stature.

Lab

- Measuring the height velocity is a sensitive indicator of growth failure.
- CBC: anemia seen in celiac disease and inflammatory bowel disease.
- Renal function, TSH, CRP.
- Karyotyping in females.
- Endomysial and gliadin antibodies.
- GH provocation tests.

Imaging

- Xray of wrist and hand for bone age
- MRI of the head if neurologic signs or sx

Rx

- GH deficiency treated with biosynthetic GH given sc daily.
- Should be managed at specialist centers.
- Other indications for GH therapy include Prader-Willi syndrome, Turner syndrome, chronic renal failure, and IUGR.
- Congenital hypothyroidism is treated with thyroxine replacement therapy; treatment of acquired hypothyroidism may not prevent short stature if diagnosed late.

9.4 Tall Stature

General Ref

- *Eur J Pediatr* 1994;153:311–316

Def

- Height > 2 standard deviations above the mean

Causes

- Familial tall stature: parents and other family members tall. This is a normal variant with normal linear growth velocities, normal bone age with normal timing, and magnitude of pubertal growth spurt.
- Nutritional: overeating and obesity in childhood leads to early growth and may result in tall stature; however, puberty is often earlier so final height may not be excessive.
- Syndromes: certain syndromes are associated with tall stature (e.g., Marfan syndrome, cerebral gigantism, homocystinuria, Klinefelter syndrome).
- Endocrine causes are rare. There is early excessive growth in CAH and precocious puberty, but early epiphyseal closure leads to final reduced height. Hyperthyroidism and true gigantism due to excess GH secretion are other causes.

9.5 Abnormal Head Growth

Normal Head Growth

- Most head growth first 2 yr of life reflects brain growth. Sutures and fontanelles open at birth; posterior fontanelle is closed by 8 wk and anterior fontanelle by 12–18 months. Sutures fused by 12 months.

Microcephaly

- Familial: calculate mid parental head percentile. Presents at birth; growth and development are normal.
- Congenital infections.
- Autosomal recessive conditions associated with developmental delay.
- Acquired: hypoxic ischemic encephalopathy, meningitis.

Macrocephaly

- Familial with normal growth and development
- Hydrocephalus: progressive or arrested, neurofibromatosis, cerebral gigantism, raised intracranial pressure, chronic subdural hematoma

Asymmetric Heads

- Head circumference increases normally but imbalance of growth rate at the coronal, sagittal, or lamboid sutures.
- Increased frequency of occipital plagiocephaly due to back-to-baby campaign.

Craniosynostosis

- Premature fusion of sutures.
- May be associated with the following syndromes: Apert Crouzon, Alexander Pfeiffer, Saethre-Chotzen.

9.6   Hypothyroidism

9.6.1 Congenital Hypothyroidism

General Ref

- *Pediatrics* 2005;116:168–173
- *J Pediatr* 2009;154:263–236
- *Am J Obstet Gynecol* 2009;201:48.e1–e4

Cause

- Thyroid dysgenesis: disorders that occur during thyroid development and include ectopic thyroid, thyroid aplasia, and thyroid hypoplasia; 1 in 4500.

- Dyshormonogenesis: an inborn error of thyroid hormone synthesis, most common cause of genetic congenital hypothyroidism, more common in consanguineous marriage, may present with a goiter.
- Iodine deficiency: most common cause worldwide; rare in United States; prevented by iodination of maternal diet.
- Central hypothyroidism: < 1% due to isolated TSH deficiency; more commonly associated with panhypopituitarism (GH and ACTH deficiency tend to manifest before hypothyroidism becomes evident).

Epidem

- Congenital hypothyroidism: 85%, sporadic
- 15% hereditary: autosomal recessive
- Incidence 1 in 4000 newborns and one of the few causes of preventable severe learning disabilities
- M:F: 1:2 and more common in twins

S+S

- Independently associated with reduced variability on FHT (*Am J Obstet Gynecol* 2009;201:48.e1–e4)
- FTT, feeding problems, prolonged jaundice, constipation, coarse faces, hoarse voice, large tongue, goiter (uncommon), developmental delay, hernia

Course

- Early dx and treatment results in intelligence within normal range for most children.

Complications

- Studies suggest increased prevalence of congenital renal and urologic anomalies in these pts (*J Pediatr* 2009;154: 263–266).

Lab

- Routine neonatal screening: Guthrie test for raised TSH levels at birth, FT4 (free T4), TSH
- Hearing test (Pendred syndrome)

Imaging

- US of thyroid gland.
- Radioiodine scan.
- Consider US to look for associated renal and urologic anomalies (*J Pediatr* 2009;154:263–266).

Rx

- Starts before 3 wk; essential to prevent learning difficulties.
- Treatment is lifelong with oral thyroxine replacement therapy.
- Dose titrated to maintain normal growth, TSH, and T4 levels.

9.6.2 Childhood (Acquired) Hypothyroidism

General Ref

- *Pediatr Rev* 2004;25:94

Cause

- Hashimoto thyroiditis.
- Irradiation of the neck (e.g., radioactive iodine to treat hyperthyroidism); 10–20% develop hypothyroidism.
- Medications: propylthiouracil, carbimazole, lithium, amiodarone.
- Iodine deficiency most common worldwide; rare in United States.

- Central hypothyroidism: tumors pressing on hypothalamus or pituitary; head trauma.
- Thyroid hormone resistance: autosomal dominant receptor binding defect.

Epidem

- Most cases are sporadic.
- Hashimoto autoimmune thyroiditis is the most common cause.
- M:F: 1:2

S+S

- Short stature, cold intolerance, dry hair and skin, bradycardia, constipation, delayed puberty, obesity, learning difficulties

Prognosis

- Good if diagnosed early; recovering lost linear growth depends on the age of initiation of therapy and duration of hypothyroidism.

Lab

- Primary (thyroid gland) hypothyroidism: low T4, low FT4, and elevated TSH.
- Secondary (pituitary) and tertiary (hypothalamus) hypothyroidism low T4 and FT4 with normal to low TSH.
- TRH (thyroid-releasing hormone) stimulation test differentiates secondary from tertiary hypothyroidism: TRH results in no change in TSH in secondary hypothyroidism but an increase TSH in tertiary hypothyroidism.
- Hashimoto: increased thyroid peroxidase antibodies, antimicrosomal antibodies, and thyroglobulin antibody titers.

Imaging

- US and thyroid scan if a nodule is present
- Xray wrist to determine bone age

Rx

- Levothyroxine: monitor FT4 and TSH level every 3–6 months.
- Goal: FT4 in mid-normal and TSH in normal range.

9.7 Hyperthyroidism

General Ref

- *J Pediatr* 2005;146:533–536
- *J Pediatr Endocrinol Metab* 2008;21:1085–1088

Cause

- Graves' disease: autoimmune thyroiditis secondary to the production of thyroid-stimulating immunoglobulins.
- Neonatal hyperthyroidism may occur in infants of mothers with Graves' disease from transplacental transfer of TSI (thyroid-stimulating immunoglobulin). Treatment is needed because potentially fatal, but resolves spontaneously with time.

Epidem

- Most common in teenage girls

S+S

- Anxiety, sweating, increased appetite, diarrhea, weight loss, tremor, tachycardia, advanced bone age, goiter, learning difficulties, behavioral problems.

- Eye signs include lid lag and retraction, exophthalmus, and ophthalmoplegia. Eyes signs less common in the pediatric population.

Lab

- Elevated T3, T4, suppressed TSH levels; antithyroid peroxisomal antibodies may be present.

Rx

- β-Blockers for symptomatic relief of tremor, anxiety, or tachycardia.
- Carbimazole or propylthiouracil interfere with thyroid hormone synthesis. Treatment is continued for 2 yr and controls thyrotoxicosis but may not resolve the eye signs.
- 40–75% relapse on discontinuing therapy.
- If relapse, rx options include:
  - Second courses of drugs.
  - Radioiodine ablation or subtotal thyroidectomy.
- Follow up for signs of hypothyroidism that may require replacement therapy.
- Large-dose iodide may be used in hyperthyroid crisis.

9.8 Hypoglycemia

General Ref

- *Pediatr Rev* 1989;11:117

Cause

- Neonates: IDDM, poor stores due to prematurity
- Increased glucose use
- Decreased glycogenolysis or gluconeogenesis (seen in inborn errors of metabolism and liver disease)
- Hyperinsulinism: IDDM, Beckwith-Weidemann syndrome
- Drugs: propranolol, insulin, isoniazid, alcohol

Pathophys

- Infants have high energy requirements and relatively poor reserves of glucose from gluconeogenesis and glycogenesis so are at high risk of hypoglycemia.

S+S

- Sweating, pallor, signs of CNS irritability, headache, seizures, and coma

Complications

- Neurologic sequelae may be permanent if hypoglycemia persists: epilepsy, learning difficulties, microcephaly.

Lab

- Confirm hypoglycemia with blood glucose.
- GH, cortisol, insulin, c-peptide, acetoacetate, 3-hydroxybutyrate, glycerol, branched chain amino acids, acylcarnitine, lactate, pyruvate.
- Urine for organic acids.
- Consider saving blood and urine for toxicology.

Rx

- IV 10% glucose 2–4 mL/kg.
- If not responding, give glucagon 0.5–1 mg im.
- Consider corticosteroids if there is a possibility of hypopituitarism or hypoadrenalism.

9.9 Obesity

General Ref

- JAMA 2002;288:1728–1732

- *Pediatrics* 2007;120:S193–S228
- *Circulation* 2005;111:1999–2012

Def

- BMI > 98th percentile for age and sex.
- Overweight is a BMI > 91st percentile for age and sex.
- BMI > 95th percentile predicts an increased risk of obesity in adulthood and abnormalities in blood lipids and blood pressure.

Cause

- Increased intake of energy-dense foods and reduced exercise.
- Exogenous causes rare and include Cushing syndrome, hypothyroidism, hypogonadotrophic, hypogonadism (Prader-Willi, Laurence, Biedl-Moon syndromes).

Epidem

- Now the most common disorder affecting children and adolescents, reflecting current epidemic; more common in low socioeconomic homes.

Pathophys

- Overnutrition accelerates growth and the onset of puberty.
- Most obese children are > 50th percentile for height.
- Exogenous causes and syndromes are associated with short stature due to a decline in growth velocity.

S+S

- Look for dysmorphic features that suggest a syndrome.
- Overeating excess fat is truncal and peripheral.
- A buffalo hump suggests an endocrine cause.
- Abdominal obesity is associated with insulin resistance (may see acanthosis nigricans), PCOS (may see signs of hirsutism), and metabolic syndrome.

- Children who are obese from overeating tend to be tall, whereas obesity from syndromes is associated with short stature.
- Blurred disc margins in pseudotumor cerebri.
- Hepatomegaly may be seen due to fatty liver.

Lab

- Consider looking for comorbidities; no consensus on routine screening labs.
- BMI > 95th percentile, fasting glucose, insulin and lipid panel.
- Despite studies showing increased prevalence vitamin D deficiency in obese children, currently insufficient evidence to recommend routine screening.

Imaging

- If clinically indicated:
  - Plain Xray: of lower extremities if slipped capital femoral epiphysis (SCFE), Blount disease suspected
  - Abdominal US: if hepatomegaly, possible fatty liver or gallbladder disease.

Complications

- SCFE, benign intracranial hypertension, obstructive sleep apnea, PCOS, DM 2, hypertension, low self-esteem, depression, teasing.
- Recent studies show an increased prevalence of vitamin D deficiency in obese children with associated increased systolic BP and decreased high-density lipoprotein-cholesterol (*J Pediatr Endocrinol Metab* 2007;20:817–823).

Rx

- No evidence that drug rx is effective in children but may be considered in any child with BMI > 98th percentile and a family motivated to make the appropriate lifestyle changes, which must be sustained.

- Goals of lifestyle changes:
  - Small gradual behavior changes.
  - Healthier eating.
  - Increase in physical activity to 30–60 min of moderate to vigorous physical activity per d.
  - Reduction in physical inactivity (TV, video games) to average 2 hr per d.
  - Maintaining baseline weight will result in fall in BMI over time as height increases.

9.10 Adrenal Insufficiency

General Ref

- *J Clin Endocrinol Metab* 2005;90:3243–3250
- *N Engl J Med* 1993;328:87–94

Cause

- Primary adrenal cortical insufficiency: Addison disease is rare in children.
- Congenital adrenal hyperplasia is the most common noniatrogenic cause.
- Secondary to chronic steroid use or hypopituitarism.

S + S

- Acute presentation in infancy: salt-losing crisis with hypotension, dehydration, hyponatremia, hyperkalemia, and circulatory collapse
- Chronic presentation in older children: lethargy, vomiting, hyperpigmentation of the gums and skin creases, growth failure

Lab

- Metabolic acidosis, low sodium, low glucose, and elevated potassium.
- Low or normal plasma cortisol, elevated ACTH (except in hypopituitarism).
- Cosyntropin test: fasting cortisol level taken, 250 μg cosyntropin (ACTH analog) given, cortisol level repeated after 30 min. An increase in cortisol by > 6 μg to > 20 μg indicates adequate adrenal reserve.
- Plasma cortisol levels remain low in both primary adrenal failure and in long-standing pituitary/hypothalamic Addison disease.

Rx

- Adrenal crisis: urgent IV fluids, glucose, and hydrocortisone.
- Long-term replacement therapy with glucocorticoids and mineralocorticoids.
- Stress-dose steroids given during illness or for operations, 3- to 5-fold increase in dose
- Pts should wear MedicAlert bracelets.

9.11   Diabetes Mellitus Type 1

General Ref

- WHO 1999 *Surveillance, Definition, Diagnosis and Classification of DM and Its Complications*
- *Diabetes Care* 2001;24:27
- *Diabet Med* 2006;23:285

Cause

- Genetic component; environmental triggers

Epidem

- Prevalence 1 in 400 to 500 in United States; 15% family hx; concordance in monozygotic twins ranges from 21–71%.

Pathophys

- Inflammatory process resulting in progressive loss of β-cell mass and thus insulin deficiency.

S+S

- Weight loss, lethargy, blurred vision, polyuria, polydipsia, polyphagia, signs of dehydration, 25% present with DKA, candidal infection.

Lab

- Ref: *Diabetes Care* 2005;28:186:
  - HbA1c every 3 months
  - Anti-islet cell antibodies, anti-insulin antibodies, anti-GAD (glutamic acid decarboxylase) antibodies
  - Fasting lipids every 5 yr if normal
  - Urine microalbumin-to-creatinine ratio annually from 10 yr of age
  - Thyroid function and celiac screen every 1–2 yr

Rx

- Ref: *Diabetes Care* 2008;31:S140:
  - Educate regarding sx of hypoglycemia.
  - Start insulin dose 0.3–0.6 U/kg per d.
- Conventional insulin therapy:
  - Requires fixed eating schedule and fixed carbohydrate amounts at meals
  - NPH insulin twice per d: before breakfast and second injection either before dinner or at bedtime plus rapid-acting insulin (lispro or aspart) or short-acting regular insulin 2–3 times per day
  - Two-thirds total daily dose (TDD) before breakfast (two-thirds NPH and one-third rapid/short acting) and one-third before dinner or bedtime (two-thirds to one-half NPH and one-third to one-half rapid/short acting)

- Basal-bolus insulin therapy:
  - Lantus or Levemir daily or twice daily and rapid-acting insulin with meals (aspart or lispro).
  - 50% TDD as Lantus or Levemir and 50% rapid acting, divided 3 times daily with meals.
  - Estimating insulin-to-carbohydrate ratio: 500/TDD gives number of grams of carbohydrates that are covered by 1 unit of rapid-acting insulin.
  - Insulin pump: continuous basal insulin (lispro/aspart) with bolus for correction and food.
  - A pilot study has shown that pramlintide to a maximum dose of 30 µg per meal may benefit some adolescents with DM 1 by decreasing postprandial hyperglycemia, HbA1c, body weight, and insulin dosage (*Pediatrics* 2009;124:1344–1347).

9.12   Diabetes Mellitus Type 2 in Childhood

General Ref

- *Lancet* 2007;369:1823
- *Diabetes Care* 2006;29:212
- *National Institute for Health and Clinical Excellence Guidelines*, 2003

Cause

- Associated with obesity, positive family hx, not prone to ketosis

Epidem

- Prevalence in United States increasing: ranges from 15–45%; more common in African Americans, Latinos, and Native Americans

S+S

- Occurring in younger age groups.
- Polyuria, nocturia, enuresis, polydipsia, polyphagia.
- Malaise, behavior changes, weakness.
- Nonclassic presentation may require 2-hr glucose tolerance test.

Complications

- Hypertension, fatty liver, dyslipidemia, nephropathy, retinopathy

Lab

- Dx based on blood glucose level:
  - Fasting blood glucose of ≥ 126 mg/dL (impaired fasting blood glucose level 100–125 mg/dL) *or*
  - Random blood glucose ≥ 200 mg/dL *or*
  - 2-hr blood glucose ≥ 200 mg/dL following an oral glucose tolerance test (impaired glucose tolerance test, 2-hr blood glucose 140–200 mg/dL)
- HbA1c (repeated every 3 months)
- Fasting lipids, LFTs, urine for microalbumin (all repeated annually)

Rx

- TLC: weight control, regular aerobic exercise, healthy diet
- Oral hypoglycemics: sulfonylureas, biguanides (metformin), thiazolidinediones, α-glucosidase inhibitors
- Insulin therapy

9.13 Calcium Metabolism Disorders

9.13.1 Hypoparathyroidism

General Ref

- *Nat Genet* 1992;1:149–152

Cause

- Infants: usually congenital; DiGeorge syndrome
- Older children: usually autoimmune; associated with Addison disease
- May occur as a complication in surgical thyroidectomy

Epidem

- Rare in childhood

S+S

- Malaise, muscle twitching and cramps, carpopedal spasm, positive Chvostek sign (contraction of upper lip induced by tapping over facial nerve)

Course

- Most children may lead normal lives but require regular medication and regular checks of serum and urine electrolytes.

Complications

- Cataract formation, soft tissue calcification. Nephrocalcinosis and nephrolithiasis may result in impaired renal function.

Lab

- Low serum calcium, low serum magnesium, raised phosphate, and normal alkaline phosphatase
- PTH level very low
- Decreased urinary calcium

Rx

- Acute symptomatic hypocalcemia
- IV 10% calcium gluconate
- Chronic hypocalcemia: oral calcium and high-dose vitamin D analogs

9.13.2 Pseudo-Hypoparathyroidism

General Ref

- *Nat Genet* 2005;37:25–27

Cause

- PTH resistance

Pathophys

- Mutation in a signaling molecule resulting in end organ resistance to the action of PTH

S+S

- Short stature, round facies, short neck, obesity, subcutaneous nodules, short fourth metacarpal, mild learning difficulties

Lab

- Increased phosphate, normal alkaline phosphatase, increased PTH, decreased urinary calcium

Rx

- Pseudopseudohypoparathyroidism: normal calcium, phosphate, and PTH with pseudohypoparathyroid phenotype

9.13.3 Hypercalcemia

General Ref

- *Am Fam Physician* 2003;67:1959
- *Lancet* 1998;352–356

Cause

- Primary and secondary hyperparathyroidism, malignancy, vitamin D toxicity, increased calcium intake, neonatal familial hypocalciuric hypercalcemia, Williams syndrome

S+S

- "Stones, bones, groans and psychic moans"
  - Stones: nephrocalcinosis due to increased urinary calcium; renal colic is a common presentation and also nephrogenic DI.
  - Bones: osteoporosis, osteitis fibrosa cystica.
  - Groans: anorexia, nausea, vomiting, abdominal pain, FTT.
  - Psychic moans: confusion, lethargy, poor concentration, coma, hypertension.

Complications

- Osteopenia, nephrocalcinosis, and nephrolithiasis; hypoparathyroidism as a complication of parathyroidectomy

Lab

- EKG shortened QT
- Serum calcium and ionized calcium high, phosphate low, elevated alkaline phosphatase
- Urine calcium-to-creatinine ratio elevated
- Albumin, electrolytes, BUN, and creatinine
- Vitamin D levels: 25-hydroxy vitamin D levels usually normal and 1,25-hydroxy vitamin D levels elevated, reflecting PTH action on the kidney

Imaging

- Kidneys, ureters, bladder, and renal US if nephrolithiasis is suspected.

- Radionuclide scans identify parathyroid adenomas.

Rx

- Vigorous hydration with normal saline.
- Diuresis: furosemide increases urinary calcium excretion.
- Restrict calcium and vitamin D intake.
- Calcitonin may provide rapid improvement, but tachyphylaxis usually develops.
- Surgical removal of a single parathyroid adenoma is usually curative.

9.13.4 Familial Hypocalciuric Hypercalcemia

General Ref

- *Nat Clin Pract Endocrinol Metab* 2007;3(2):122–133
- *Ann Intern Med* 1985;102(4):511–519

Cause

- Inherited autosomal dominant disorder

Pathophys

- Disorder of calcium-sensing receptor resulting in a higher set point for serum calcium

S+S

- Most pts asymptomatic

Course

- Benign asymptomatic condition

Lab

- Low to normal urinary calcium; PTH is normal or elevated.

Rx

- Treatment unnecessary

Chapter 10
Adolescence

10.1 Polycystic Ovary Syndrome

General Ref

- *N Engl J Med* 2005;325:1223
- *Endocrinol Metabol Clin North Am* 2005;34:677
- *J Clin Endocrinol Metab* 2009;94:1579

Cause

- Low levels of circulating progestins cause increased activity of pulsatile gonadotropin-releasing hormone, increased levels of LH, and increased ovarian androgen production.

Epidem

- Of 5–10% of women affected, 50–75% are obese.

Pathophys

- Visceral adiposity associated with hyperandrogenemia, insulin resistance, glucose intolerance, and dyslipidemia

S+S

- Acne, hirsutism, male pattern baldness, acanthosis nigricans

Course

- Untreated PCOS: increased risk of cardiovascular disease, type 2 DM, endometrial cancer, hyperlipidemia, myocardial infarction, and stroke

Complications

- Associated with hyperlipidemia, endometrial cancer, early cardiovascular disease

Lab

- Rotterdam Criteria 2003: two-thirds of individuals with oligomenorrhea or amenorrhea and hyperandrogenism have radiographic evidence of PCOS.
- Elevated LH: FSH ratio, decreased sex hormone-binding globulin (SHBG), fasting lipids, abnormal glucose tolerance test.

Imaging

- Pelvic and adrenal US. Polycystic appearance of ovaries not diagnostic (8–25% of normal women may have similar appearance).

Rx

- Weight loss, regular exercise, healthy diet improve cardiovascular status.
- Metformin improves glucose tolerance.
- Combined oral contraceptives improve hyperandrogenism, protect the endometrium from hyperplasia, protect against osteoporosis, and may improve lipid profile.
- Spironolactone has an antiandrogen effect.

10.2   Menstrual Disorders

General Ref

- *Adolesc Med State Art Rev* 2003;14:289

10.2.1 Dysmenorrhea

Cause

- Primary due to prostaglandin production by secretory endometrium

- Secondary due to polyps, fibroids, endometriosis, pelvic in-flammatory disease, adhesions, ovarian mass

Epidem

- Most common adolescent menstrual problem. Affects up to 60% postmenarchal adolescents 12–17 yr of age

Pathophys

- Primary: increased prostaglandin production by secretory endometrium resulting in myometrial contractions

S+S

- Crampy abdominal pain during menses, nausea, vomiting, backache, bloating, diarrhea.
- Primary: usually family hx; starts once ovulatory cycles occur and worst in first 2–3 d.
- Secondary: occurs immediately with menarche; pain is unusually severe or increasing in intensity.

Lab

- Primary: no tests usually needed
- Secondary: CBC, ESR, pelvic US, diagnostic laparoscopy in severe pain to r/o endometriosis

Rx

- Primary: NSAIDs (e.g., ibuprofen, naproxen, mefenamic acid) act by inhibiting synthesis and action of prostaglandins.
- If no improvement, consider workup for secondary causes.

10.2.2 Dysfunctional Uterine Bleeding

Def

- Menorrhagia: heavy bleeding occurring during normally timed cycles

- Polymenorrhea: normal flow at decreased intervals between cycles
- Metrorrhagia: heavy bleeding at irregular intervals
- Dysfunctional uterine bleeding (DUB): painless, abnormal bleeding pattern from an immature hypothalamic-pituitary-ovarian (HPO) axis, without illness or structural defect. There may be menorrhagia or metrorrhagia; dx of exclusion.

Cause

- Immature HPO axis resulting in impairment of normal negative feedback resulting in an excessively thickened endometrium that sheds once it becomes unstable, resulting in prolonged heavy bleeding.

S+S

- Irregular cycles
- Heavy bleeding; usually painless
- Prolonged bleeding > 10 d
- If severe, weakness, headaches, lightheadedness, fatigue

Lab

- CBC with differential, ESR, TSH
- Pregnancy test, gonorrhea and chlamydia probe, and wet prep if sexually active
- Coagulation screen: PT, PTT, BT, von Willebrand factor
- FSH, LH, prolactin, and serum androgens

Imaging

- Pelvic US

Rx

- Depends on degree of anemia.
- Hgb > 12 g/dL without active bleeding: reassure and treat with prophylactic iron supplementation. Follow up in 3 months.

- Hgb 10–12g/dL with active bleeding: low-dose monophasic combined oral contraceptives 2–4 times daily until the bleeding stops; taper over 21 d; iron supplements.
- Hgb 10–12g/dL with no bleeding: low-dose monophasic oral contraceptives daily for 3–6 months; iron supplements.
- Hb < 10g/dL with active bleeding:
  - Admit if hemodynamically unstable and consider transfusion.
  - Conjugated estrogens 25 mg IV every 4 hr until bleeding slows with high-dose combined oral contraceptives every 6 hr until bleeding stops.
  - If bleeding continues, do a pelvic US and consider D + C.
  - Then taper to 1 tablet 3 times daily for 3 d, twice daily for 2 wk, then daily for 1 cycle. Switch to low-dose oral contraceptives for 3–6 months and give iron supplements.

10.2.3 Amenorrhea

Def

- Primary amenorrhea: normal breast and pubic hair development with absence of menses by 16 yr or no menses by age 14 yr with no development of breast or pubic hair. Mean time between onset of breast development and puberty is 2 yr.
- Secondary amenorrhea: previously normal cycles with absence of menses for more than 6 months or 3 previous cycles.
- Cause: pregnancy; hypo- and hyperthyroidism; disorders of the hypothalamus, pituitary, or ovaries; obesity; eating disorders; chronic disease; androgen excess: PCOS.

Pathophys

- Hypothalamic and pituitary disorders present with low LH and FSH (hypogonadotrophic hypogonadism).

- High levels of gonadotropins suggest ovarian failure (hyper-gonadotrophic hypogonadism).

S+S

- Absence of menses
- Primary: assess the following:
  - Stage of breast and pubic hair development
  - Family hx, diet and exercise hx, BMI
  - Patency of vagina
  - Signs of virilization: acne, hirsutism, clitoromegaly (PCOS)
  - Stigmata of syndromes (e.g., Turner syndrome, Prader-Willi syndrome)
- Secondary: assess the following:
  - Stress level, weight changes, exercise hx
  - Sexual hx
  - Headaches, visual changes
  - Galactorrhea
  - Signs of virilization

Lab

- Primary:
  - CBC, ESR, TSH, bone age.
  - Consider chemistry panel and UA if systemic illness suspected.
  - If short stature: abdominal US to assess presence of uterus (must be done before considering medroxyprogesterone challenge); if absent, karyotyping to differentiate testicular feminization syndrome from müllerian duct defect.
  - If no withdrawal bleeding with medroxyprogesterone challenge, check FSH, LH, and prolactin.
  - Low levels of gonadotropins suggest hypothalamic suppression; high levels suggest ovarian failure or gonadal dysgenesis.
  - Consult endocrinology.

- Secondary:
  - Pregnancy test.
  - If signs of virilization, check LH:FSH ratio ($> 2.5:1$ commonly seen in PCOS), free testosterone, 17-hydorxyprogesterone; DHEAS levels to help differentiate PCOS from androgen-producing ovarian or adrenal tumors.
  - If negative pregnancy test, progesterone challenge as for primary:
    - Withdrawal flow in 1–2 wk suggests sufficient estrogen.
  - Check LH:
    - High LH suggests PCOS.
    - Low or normal LH: Check prolactin and TSH level:
      - High TSH and prolactin: hypothyroidism and treat accordingly.
      - Normal TSH high prolactin: MRI of head to r/o prolactinoma.
      - Normal prolactin: mild hypothalamic suppression due to weight changes, stress, illness, strenuous exercise.
  - No withdrawal bleeding or withdrawal bleeding followed by continued amenorrhea suggests inadequate estrogen levels:
    - Check FSH levels:
      - High FSH suggests premature ovarian failure (e.g., autoimmune, secondary to chemotherapy)
      - Low or normal FSH: MRI of head to r/o out brain tumor (e.g., craniopharyngioma).

Rx

- Primary:
  - If pelvic organs and external genitalia are normal, challenge with medroxyprogesterone (MP):
    - MP 10 mg po twice daily for 5 d or 10 mg daily for 7–10 d.
    - Withdrawal bleeding within 7 d implies normal anatomy and adequate estrogen effect.

- Secondary:
  - Treat the cause.
  - Thyroid replacement in hypothyroidism.
  - Birth control pills and consider metformin in PCOS.
  - Ovarian failure: consult gynecology or endocrinology.
  - Severe hypothalamic dysfunction: consult neurology.
  - Adrenal or androgen problems: consult endocrinology.

10.3 Infectious Mononucleosis

General Ref

- *J Infect Dis* 2007;196:4
- *Clin J Sport Med* 2005;15:410–416

Cause

- The herpes virus EBV

Epidem

- Humans are the only reservoirs; transmitted through respiratory secretions and sexual activity in adolescents. Incubation period: 30–50 d.

S+S

- Young children with EBV often asymptomatic; older children: fever, malaise, anorexia
- Pharyngitis that may be exudative, palatial petechiae, tender cervical lymphadenopathy, splenomegaly, hepatomegaly

Course

- Usually benign.
- Some pts have persisting fatigue and malaise several months after infection.

Complications

- Splenic rupture (a rare complication)
- Aseptic meningitis, encephalitis
- Bell palsy, Guillain-Barré syndrome

Lab

- CBC and differential: atypical lymphocytosis (leukopenia may occur early).
- Elevated amylase.
- Positive heterophile antibodies (positive in > 90% adults but < 50% children < 5 yr).
- EBV PCR used for dx in CNS and ocular infections.

Rx

- Supportive: bed rest; acetaminophen for fever.
- Avoid contact sports if splenomegaly. Consensus evidence for safety to return to sport includes pt being asymptomatic, afebrile, well hydrated, with no hepatomegaly or splenomegaly (*Clin J Sport Med* 2005;15:410–416).

10.4   Pelvic Inflammatory Disease

General Ref

- Center for Disease Control and Prevention, *Sexually Transmitted Infections Treatment Guidelines*, 2006.
- *MMWR Recomm Rep* 2006;55(RR-11):1–94
- www.cdc.gov/std/treatment

Cause

- Usually polymicrobial. *Neisseria gonorrhea* and *Chlamydia* most common organisms; also *Haemophilus* influenza and anaerobes

Epidem

- Adolescent girls account for 20–30% of all cases; affects > 1 million women per yr in United States

Pathophys

- Direct ascending spread of bacteria to the upper female genital tract in sexually active individual.

S+S

- Gradual onset of bilateral or unilateral, mild to moderate lower abdominal pain.
- Pain is aggravated by movement (PID shuffle: slow careful gait to avoid sudden movement that increases peritoneal irritation).
- Dyspareunia, anorexia, nausea, vomiting.
- Pelvic examination:
    - Cervical motion tenderness, adnexal fullness and tenderness.
    - Positive Chandelier sign: pt lifts the body away from examiner.
    - Fever, mucopurulent vaginal discharge.

Course

- Complications: tubo-ovarian abscess, perihepatitis (Fitz-Hugh-Curtis syndrome), infertility due to tubal occlusion (infertility risk increases with recurrent infection)

Lab

- CBC; elevated WCC with left shift.
- ESR and CRP elevated.
- Swabs for gonorrhea and chlamydia testing.
- Wet prep.
- Consider syphilis serology.

- HIV testing (counseling and follow-up important).

Imaging

- Transvaginal pelvic US to r/o tubo-ovarian abscess
- Abdominal CT scan if abscess suspected

Rx

- CDC has devised criteria for rx of PID.
- Minimum criteria/recommendations as follows:
  - Empirical treatment of PID should be initiated in sexually active young women at risk of STIs if the following minimum criteria are met and no other cause is found for illness: uterine or adnexal tenderness (*Red Book* 2009).
  - Previously inpt management was recommended for all adolescents with PID; there are no data supporting this approach.
  - Outpt antibiotic treatment is appropriate if sx are not severe; no concerns re tubo-ovarian abscess, ectopic pregnancy, or appendicitis; and pt is reliable and compliant with treatment.
- CDC treatment regimens (*Red Book* 2009):
  - Outpt management ambulatory regimen:
    - Ceftriaxone 250 mg im once *or* cefoxitin 2 g im and probenecid 1 g po concurrently once *or* other parenteral third-generation cephalosporins *plus* doxycycline 100 mg po twice daily for 14 d *with or without* metronidazole 500 mg po twice daily for 14 d
  - Inpt management:
    - Parenteral regimen A: cefotetan 2 g IV twice daily *or* cefoxitin 2 g IV 4 times daily *plus* doxycycline 100 mg po or IV twice daily for 14 d
    - Parenteral regimen B: clindamycin 900 mg IV 3 times daily *plus* gentamicin loading dose IV or im 2 mg/kg followed by maintenance 1.5 mg/kg 3 times daily or daily

- May stop parenteral therapy 24 hr after clinical improvement and change to doxycycline 100 mg po twice daily or clindamycin 450 mg po 4 times daily for 14 d

10.5 Eating Disorders

General Ref

- *Curr Probl Pediatr* 1995;25:67–89
- MMWR Surveill Summ 2008;57(4):1–113
- Diagnostic criteria (*DSM-IV*) for anorexia nervosa:
  - Self-induced weight loss > 15% below ideal body weight
  - Amenorrhea in postpubertal females
  - Intense fear of weight gain despite being underweight
  - Abnormal perception of body image
- Diagnostic criteria (*DSM-IV*) for bulimia nervosa:
  - Uncontrollable binge eating
  - Repeated inappropriate behavior to try and prevent weight gain (e.g., self-induced vomiting, laxative abuse)
  - Behaviors just described occur at least twice a wk for 3 months
  - Overly concerned with body shape and weight

Cause

- Familial factors: concordance rate for anorexia nervosa 50% in monozygotic twins versus 10% in dizygotic twins (*Am J Psychiatry* 1991;148:1627–1637)
- Socioeconomic factors: social pressures, sports that emphasize leanness (e.g., gymnastics)

Epidem

- Increasing incidence over last 20 yr.
- Rare in prepubertal children; most common in mid and late adolescence.

- More than 90% affected are female.

S+S

- Hx: weight changes, changes in sleep pattern, excessive exercise, fatigue, syncope or presyncopal episodes, constipation, dieting, purging, laxative or diuretic abuse.
- Physical exam: look for signs of purging (e.g., enlarged parotid, soft palate lesions, knuckle calluses, dental erosions) (*Arch Intern Med* 2005;165(5):561–566).

Course

- Mortality in anorexia nervosa 10 times that of the general population; cardiac dysrhythmia and suicide most common causes.
- 50% recover completely; 25% partial recovery with recurrences; 25% no improvement.

Complications

- Osteopenia, cardiac dysrhythmias, amenorrhea

Lab

- CBC and differential, electrolytes, BUN, and creatinine
- ESR routinely low to normal
- Glucose, calcium, magnesium, phosphorous, UA
- TSH, T3, and T4
- Prolactin, FSH, pregnancy test
- EKG
- Bone densitometry (DEXA scan) indicated if pt presents with fractures or amenorrhea for > 6 months

Rx

- Requires a multidisciplinary team approach.
- Nutritional rehabilitation: American Psychiatric Association has established guidelines for treatment (*Am J Psychiatry* 2006;163[Suppl 1]:1).

- Psychotherapy: cognitive behavior therapy most effective in bulimia nervosa (*Am J Psychiatry* 1997;154:523–531); efficacy not so clear for anorexia nervosa.
- Medication: limited role in anorexia nervosa. High-dose fluoxetine 40–80 mg/d demonstrated to decrease bingeing and purging (*Br J Psychiatry* 1995;166:660–666).
- Society of Adolescent Medicine has published guidelines for hospitalization (*J Adolesc Health* 2003;33:496).

Chapter 11

Cardiology

11.1 Heart Murmurs

Cause

- Turbulent blood flow through heart or great vessels. Incidence as high as 75%. Most murmurs nonpathologic; however, they can be indicator of heart disease.
- Auscultation should occur *after* inspection, palpation of precordium/pulses/skin perfusion/abdomen.
- Consult pediatric cardiologist; echocardiogram is defining test but should be directed by specialist.

Types

- Innocent murmurs: Still disease—musical, vibratory, hooting mid systolic, left lower sternal border (LLSB), decreases in intensity when sits. Basal flow murmur—crescendo-decrescendo murmur due to blood flowing out of the pulmonary artery (PA) or aorta. Peripheral pulmonic stenosis—turbulence in the branching of the PA causes flow murmur that radiates to the axillae; venous hums—typically louder in diastole and blowing; suppressed by lying down or jugular compression. Bruits common in normals.
- Pathologic murmurs variably difficult to recognize. Ventricular septal defect typically leads to a blowing holosystolic noise at LLSB (obscures S1). Atrial septal defect more subtle; fixed splitting of S2 is the key to dx. Aortic valvular stenosis and

pulmonary valvular stenosis can be subtle, but the association with systolic clicks helps sort them from normal.

11.2   Cardiac Arrhythmias

11.2.1 Supraventricular Tachycardia

General Ref

- *Pediatr Clin North Am* 2006;53:85

Cause

- Most cases are idiopathic.
- Associated with myocarditis, Wolff-Parkinson-White (WPW) syndrome, congenital heart disease (Ebstein anomaly, transposition of the great vessels).
- Precipitants include exercise, drugs, fever, infection.

Epidem

- Most common childhood arrhythmia.
- 50–60% of children present in the 1st yr of life.

Pathophys

- Reentry tachycardia, circuit of conduction with premature activation of the atrium via an accessory pathway.

S+S

- Infants may present with poor feeding, diaphoresis, irritability. Toddlers and older children may have syncope, shortness of breath, palpitations, chest pain.

Course

- May recur.
- Infants usually on prophylaxis 1st yr of life then observed off treatment.

- Frequent recurrence: consider radiofrequency ablation.

Lab

- EKG shows narrow complex tachycardia at a rate of 250–300 bpm.

Imaging

- Chest Xray: may show cardiomegaly if heart failure

Rx

- Assess ABCs.
- If hemodynamically stable, initiate the following:
  - Vagal maneuvers.
  - Adenosine IV 50–300 µg/kg per dose.
- If hemodynamically unstable:
  - DC synchronized cardioversion 0.5–2 J/kg.
  - Prophylaxis: flecainide, sotalol, propranolol, digoxin (contraindicated in WPW syndrome).
  - Radiofrequency catheter ablation is an alternative to long-term drug therapy.

11.2.2 Congenital Heart Block

General Ref

- *Pediatrics* 1982;69:728–733

Cause

- Associated with maternal SLE and the presence of anti-Ro or anti-La antibodies in maternal serum
- Following corrected transposition of the great vessels (TGV)

Pathophys

- Anti- Ro and anti-La antibodies prevent normal development of the electrical conduction system of the developing heart with resultant atrophy and fibrosis of the atrioventricular node (AVN).

S+S

- In utero death, fetal hydrops
- Present at birth with heart rate 70 bpm and are usually well
- Often no treatment required for yr
- If resting heart rate < 40 bpm, may present with FTT, collapse, Stokes-Adams attacks, and heart failure

Course

- Most remain asymptomatic for yr.

Rx

- All symptomatic children require endocardial pacemaker placement.
- Follow up with 24-hr EKG every 2–3 months.

11.2.3 Long QT Syndrome

General Ref

- *Ann Intensive Med* 2002;137:981–992

Cause

- Congenital forms:
  - Romano-Ward: nonlethal autosomal dominant
  - Jervell and Lange-Nielsen autosomal recessive: associated with sensorineural hearing loss
  - Other associations: hypocalcemia, hypokalemia, hypomagnesemia, head injury and hypothermia, erythromycin and cisapride

S+S

- Onset late childhood
- Sudden loss of consciousness following stress, exercise, or emotion
- If unrecognized, may result in sudden death from ventricular tachycardia

Lab

- EKG

11.2.4 Others

- Atrial fibrillation, flutter, ectopic atrial tachycardia, ventricular fibrillation all rare in childhood and more common in children who have had surgery for complex cardiac conditions.

11.3 Syncope

General Ref

- *J Am Coll Cardiol* 1997;29:1039–1045
- *J Pediatr* 2004;145:223–228

Cause

- Dehydration, fatigue, prolonged standing, hypoglycemia, watching venipuncture

Epidem

- 20–50% will have a vasovagal episode by 20 yr of age.

Pathophys

- Cerebral ischemia causing a transient loss of consciousness and postural tone

S+S

- Dizziness, nausea, pallor, diaphoresis; may be associated with brief tonic-clonic seizures

Course

- Benign; avoid precipitants. If secondary cause, prognosis depends on the cause.

CARDIOLOGY

Lab

- EEG normal
- May have autonomic dysfunction with exaggerated orthostatic hypotension
- If recurrent episodes: CBC, glucose, electrolytes, Holter monitoring

Rx

- Look for and avoid precipitating factors.
- Ensure adequate salt and fluid intake.

11.4   Hypertension

General Ref

- *J Pediatr* 2006;148:195–200
- *J Vasc Surg* 2005;41:973–982

Definition

- Average systolic and/or diastolic BPs > 95th percentile for gender and age

Cause

- Usually secondary causes in childhood.
- Renal: tumors—Wilms, renovascular—renal artery stenosis, renal parenchymal disease
- Excess catecholamines: phaeochromocytoma, neuroblastoma
- Endocrine: congenital adrenal hyperplasia (CAH), Cushing syndrome
- Cardiac: coarctation of the aorta
- Essential: positive family hx, obesity

Epidem

- Infants: secondary and congenital causes more common; adolescents: essential more common

Pathophys

- Depends on the cause

S+S

- Headache, vomiting, facial palsy, convulsions, FTT, paroxysmal palpitations and sweating in phaeochromocytoma

Lab

- Ambulatory BP measurements
- UA, serum electrolytes, creatinine, BUN
- Calcium, cholesterol, uric acid, CBC
- Further studies guided by clinical picture (e.g., plasma catecholamines and metanephrines)

Imaging

- Echocardiogram (to monitor end organ damage)
- Renal US
- Further imaging guided by clinical picture (e.g., DMSA renal scan, MCUG)

Rx

- Mild essential hypertension: control weight, regular exercise, sodium restriction
- Renal cause: angiotensin converting enzyme inhibitor (ACEI)
- Essential: vasodilators, diuretics, and β-blockers
- Surgery: nephrectomy in unilateral scarring, repair of coarctation, resection of a phaeochromocytoma
- Angioplasty for renal artery stenosis
- Dialysis for chronic renal failure

CARDIOLOGY

Chapter 12
Rheumatology

12.1 Juvenile Idiopathic Arthritis

General Ref

- *Rheumatology (Oxford)* 2002;41(12):1428–1435
- *J Rheumatol* 2008;35(2):343–348
- *Lancet* 2007;369:767

Cause

- Heterogenous group of chronic arthritides affecting one or more joints, occurring for at least 6 wk, pt < 16 yr. Dx of exclusion. Cause unknown but a genetic predisposition, autoimmunity, and possibly infection are all thought to play a role.

Epidem

- Age of onset < 16 yr; 70,000–100,000 children affected per yr in the United States

Pathophys

- Chronic synovial inflammation of unknown etiology

S+S

- Depending on the type:
  - Systemic: 9% of JIA, age of onset 1–10 yr; M:F

- Clinical presentation: daily fever spikes for up to 2 wk; maculopapular salmon pink rash with one or more of the following: hepatomegaly, splenomegaly, pericarditis, lymphadenopathy, serositis. Arthritis maybe absent at the onset. May have myalgia or arthralgia. Arthritis is oligoarticular or polyarticular. ESR, WCC, and platelets are all elevated; normochromic normocytic anemia. Half have recurrent episodes; one-third have progressive arthritis. Amyloidosis with renal failure is a rare but serious complication:
- Oligoarticular persistent: 49%; age of onset 1–6 yr, M:F: 1:5
  - Clinical presentation: ≤ 4 joints involved; affected limb has accelerated growth so leg length discrepancy may be seen, most commonly knees, ankle, or wrist; 60–70% ANA positive, increased risk of chronic iridocyclitis, associated with HLA DR5. Restricted to ≤ 4 joints after 6 months. Excellent prognosis.
- Oligoarticular extended: 8%; ≤ 4 joints but extends to > 4 joints after 6 months. Otherwise similar presentation to the persistent form except prognosis more guarded.
- Polyarticular RF negative: 16%, age of onset 1–6 yr, M:F: 1:5
  - Clinical presentation: ≥ 5 joints involving both large and small joints. TMJ (temporomandibular joint) and cervical spine maybe involved; occasional low-grade fever; 5% chronic anterior uveitis. ESR, WCC, platelets are all increased, RF negative, ANA positive, normochromic, normocytic anemia. Prognosis is variable.
- Polyarticular RF positive: 3%; ≥ 5 joints involved, age of onset 10–16 yr; M:F: 1:5
  - Clinical presentation: symmetric large and small joint involvement with marked finger involvement,

rheumatoid nodules at pressure points. Increased ESR, WCC, and platelets; RF positive and ANA positive; HLADR4 positive. Prognosis is poor.

- Psoriatic arthritis: 7%; age of onset 1–16 yr; M:F
  - Clinical presentation: asymmetric involvement of large and small joints; scaly rash may coincide with arthritis; nail pitting, dactylitis of fingers and toes typical; DIP (distal interphalangeal) involvement typical. May develop uveitis. There may be a family hx of psoriasis and may be ANA positive. Prognosis is moderate.
- Enthesitis related: 7%; age of onset 6–16 yr; M:F: 4:1
  - Clinical presentation: initially lower limb, large joint involvement, with later involvement of lumbar and sacroiliac spine. Enthesitis: localized inflammation of tendon or ligament insertions. Occasional acute uveitis. Prognosis is moderate. HLA B27 positive.
  - Undifferentiated arthritis: 1%; age of onset 1–16 yr; M:F: 1:2. Overlapping articular and extra-articular patterns between 2 or more subtypes. Prognosis variable.

Complications

- Chronic anterior uveitis is asymptomatic and may lead to visual impairment. Regular slit lamp exam screening indicated especially in oligoarticular subtypes.
- Flexion contractures.
- Chronic disease may lead to joint destruction and the need for joint replacement.
- Growth failure maybe secondary to chronic disease, anorexia, and steroid therapy.
- Amyloidosis: rare but serious complication in systemic form.

Lab

- ESR, WCC, platelets, ANA, RF

Xray

- Xray may be initially normal; helps exclude trauma and other bony lesions.
- US helpful in identifying an effusion. US-guided joint aspiration for culture and sensitivity.
- Bone scan, MRI useful to identify osteomyelitis.

Rx

- Requires a multidisciplinary approach to management.
- Goal to maintain quality of life and preserve joint function.
- NSAIDs in all children with active disease to control pain and suppress inflammation.
- Intra-articular corticosteroids may be helpful. Systemic steroids avoided due to side effects but may be needed in severe polyarticular or systemic disease.
- Disease-modifying antirheumatic drugs used if no response to the above. Methotrexate most widely used sc or po.
- Anti-TNF therapy: etanercept if not well controlled on methotrexate.

12.2   Systemic Lupus Erythematosus

General Ref

- *N Engl J Med* 2008;358:929
- *J Pediatr* 2005;146:648–653

Cause

- Prototype autoimmune disease; etiology unknown. Triggers include EBV, parvovirus B19.

Epidem

- Uncommon in pts < 5 yr.

- Prevalence increases during adolescence and adulthood.
- M:F: 1:9.
- Affects Afro-Caribbeans, African Americans, and Asians more than whites.

Pathophys

- Polygenic disease. Family members are commonly ANA positive and have another autoimmune disease.

S+S

- Criteria for dx is ≥ 4 of the following (*J Pediatr* 2005;146:648):
  - Malar rash
  - Discoid rash
  - Photosensitivity
  - Oral ulcers
  - Nonerosive arthritis in ≥ 1 joint
  - Serositis (involvement of the pleura or pericardium)
  - Renal disease: persistent proteinuria, granular casts
  - Neurologic disorder: seizures, psychosis (*J Rheumatol* 2002;29:1536–1542)
  - Hematologic disorder: hemolytic anemia, leukopenia, lymphopenia, thrombocytopenia
  - Immunologic disorder: APA positive, anti-DNA antibodies, anti–smooth muscle antibodies, false-positive VDRL, ANA positive

Course

- 90% 10-yr survival; renal involvement and hypertension have a worse prognosis.
- Premature death associated with atherosclerosis and stroke.
- Risk factors for poor outcome: noncompliance, poor socioeconomic status, and cognitive deterioration.

RHEUMATOLOGY

Lab

- CBC, ESR
- Renal bx
- ANA, anti–smooth muscle, anti–double-stranded DNA antibodies, anti-Ro, anti-La
- VDRL, complement levels

Rx

- Psychosocial support.
- Provide photoprotection.
- Mild disease with no renal involvement:
    - NSAIDS, hydroxychloroquine 7 mg/kg per day to maximum of 400 mg; low-dose steroids often necessary to maintain control.
    - Moderate disease: often need high-dose steroids, methotrexate and/or azathioprine can be used for steroid-sparing effect.
- Severe disease: with substantial renal or neurologic involvement:
    - Monthly IV pulses of cyclophosphamide (500 mg/m^2 increasing to 1 g/m^2 as tolerated) for 6 months, followed by every 3 months cyclophosphamide for an additional 30 months.
    - Other:
        - Mycophenolate: Children with renal disease resistant to other immunosuppressive agents may benefit from treatment with mycophenolate mofetil (*J Rheumatol* 2001;28:2103–2108).
        - Rituximab: a chimeric anti-CD20 monoclonal antibody; has been used effectively, often in combination with cyclophosphamide, in the treatment of children with severe SLE refractory to conventional therapy (*Arch Dis Child* 2008;93:401).

- Stem cell transplantation: advocated for children with severe SLE; however, unlikely to be widely used due to significant associated morbidity and mortality (*Lupus* 2004;13:89–94).

12.3   Acute Rheumatic Fever

General Ref

- JAMA 1992;268:2069–2073
- *Lancet Infect Dis* 2005;5:685–694

Cause

- Abnormal immune response to a preceding infection with beta-hemolytic strep group A

Pathophys

- Autoimmune theories: cross-reacting antibodies; humans and strep share antigen. Only strep pharyngitis causes acute rheumatic fever (ARF), so other mechanism likely involved.

Epidem

- Peak incidence: 5–15 yr of age
- M:F: 3:1
- Marked decrease with the widespread use of penicillin

S+S

- Latent period of 2–6 wk following a pharyngeal infection
- Fever, malaise, polyarthritis
- Diagnostic criteria/Jones criteria:
  - Two major or 1 major plus 2 minor, plus positive antistreptolysin-O titer (ASOT) or culture or hx of scarlet fever
  - Major criteria: carditis, polyarthritis, erythema marginatum, subcutaneous nodules, chorea

RHEUMATOLOGY

- Minor criteria: fever, polyarthralgia, increased WCC, raised acute phase reactants: ESR or CRP, prolonged PR interval or other EKG abnormalities

Course

- 10–12 wk in 80–90%.
- 95% have murmurs within 2 wk of onset.
- Severity of rheumatic heart disease is associated with the number of episodes of rheumatic fever in childhood.
- High risk of recurrence in pt who do not receive adequate prophylaxis against strep infection.

Complications

- Chronic valvular heart disease, transient glomerulonephritis

Lab

- CBC, elevated ESR, elevated ASO
- EKG: prolonged PR interval

Xray

- Chest Xray: interstitial pneumonitis.
- Echocardiogram may show valvular or myocardial dysfunction.

Rx

- Acute episode managed with bed rest and anti-inflammatories.
- High-dose aspirin is effective in suppressing the inflammatory response in the heart and joints. If no response, steroids indicated.
- Prophylaxis following resolution of acute episode:
  - Penicillin V 250 mg po twice daily in adults or daily in children or benzathine penicillin im monthly; most effective.
  - Erythromycin is used in penicillin allergy.
- Prophylaxis had been recommended until 18–21 yr of age, but recent recommendations are for lifelong prophylaxis.

Chapter 13

Psychiatric Conditions

13.1 Attention Deficit Hyperactivity Disorder

General Ref

- *Pediatrics* 2000;105:1158–1170, AAP Evaluation Guidelines
- *Pediatrics* 2001;108:1033–1044, AAP Treatment Guidelines
- *Pediatrics* 2004;113:754–776, MTA Study
- *Pediatric Annals* 2008;37(1), entire issue
- *N Engl J Med* 2005;352(2):165–172

Def

- Most common neuropsychiatric condition of childhood, characterized by deficits in the domain of inattention/focusing and/or hyperactivity/impulsivity

Pathophys

- Thought to be a genetically transmitted problem stemming from neurophysiologic imbalance rather than behavioral or psychodynamic etiology

Epidem

- Current cross-cultural studies show 3–5% prevalence globally. Higher male prevalence; females have higher proportion of inattentive subtype.
- Dx typically made in school-age children, although recent increase in preschool dx.

Dx

- AAP guidelines outline current standard of care. Gather information from multiple sources, especially teachers and parents; impairment should be noted in multiple settings. Diagnostic criteria specify that sx have been noted before age 7 yr.
- Dx includes *DSM* criteria and behavioral questionnaires (AAP Vanderbilt forms); screening questions for oppositional behaviors, anxiety, and so on; items to estimate degree of impairment.
- The dx interview is also important to catalog current or potential psychiatric comorbidities (learning disabilities, anxiety, depression, oppositional defiant disorder [ODD], conduct disorder, enuresis, encopresis, tic disorder, sleep disorder, sensory issues, explosive behavior).

Physical Exam

- Typically normal, although child may demonstrate impulsivity and intrusive speech even in the office setting.
- Exam should focus on complicating medical conditions: document normal vision and hearing; oral exam for untreated caries or tonsilloadenoidal hypertrophy suggesting possible obstructive sleep apnea syndrome (OSAS); cardiac exam to assure no unrecognized congenital heart defect that would increase theoretical risk of stimulants; abdominal exam for stool retention.

Lab

- None recommended, although consider EKG before starting stimulants.
- AAP considers careful H+P adequate for cardiac screening.

Indications for Rx

- *DSM*-based questionnaires map out elements in both domains of inattention and hyperactivity; 6 of 9 positive responses in either or both domains, with documentation of impairment in multiple settings, suggest need for rx.

- If diagnostic interview uncovers multiple comorbid diagnoses, consider referral to specialty center for complete diagnostic profile before initiating rx.

Using Stimulants

- The MTA study demonstrated that medications are more effective in alleviating core ADHD sx than behavioral interventions. The other finding from the study is that careful dose titration improves outcome.
- AAP guidelines recommend initiating treatment with one stimulant, titrating dose, and watching for side effects. About 80% of pts respond to this technique. Side effects include abdominal discomfort or headache; interference with appetite and sleep. Titration based on effect, not weight. ADHD is a lifelong condition. Frequent visits to monitor HR, BP, and weight along with sx scores are useful for maintaining compliance. Currently no established limits for HR and BP changes allowed; cardiac consultation may be useful for reassurance.
- Stimulant preparations vary both by class and by kinetics. Some children respond to short-acting preparations; others have better response (or fewer side effects) to time-released formulations. Some children show higher levels of stimulant tolerance.

Alternatives to Stimulants

- Most commonly used nonstimulant medication is atomoxetine, a norepinephrine uptake inhibitor marketed and approved for ADHD. Alpha-agonists have also been used, more typically to decrease hyperactivity and aggression than to improve attention. Bupropion is thought to have some activity against core sx. Titrating nonstimulant medications are more challenging; may take wk after initiation to see maximal effect.

Tics and Stimulants

- Tic disorders are frequently present with ADHD; some children carry Tourette's dx. Presence of tics is not contraindication to stimulant rx; tics may come and go in the absence of pharmacologic exposure, although baseline may increase in some children on stimulants. Clinician and family should assess if improvement in ADHD sx balances exacerbation of the tic. Pharmacotherapy for tics is unsatisfactory.

ADHD and Mental Retardation

- Children with mild MR can have comorbid ADHD and generally do well on stimulants.
- Autism spectrum disorders:
  - Not a contraindication to stimulants. Behavioral sx in this context are notoriously difficult to categorize; however, and the impulsivity or inattention may have an alternative etiology. Caution should be applied if medications are used because associated anxiety and "sensory issues" may be exacerbated by stimulants.

Goals of Therapy

- Increased volume and quality of academic output, decrease disruptive behavior, increased self-esteem, increased independence, enhanced safety. Long-term studies show decreased substance abuse issues, motor vehicle accidents.

13.2   Anxiety

General Ref

- www.adaa.org

- *Pediatr Ann* 36(9):586–597, pharmacotherapy for anxiety disorder
- *Gen Psychiatry* 2004;61(11):1153–1162

Def

- Anxiety disorder refers to a wide spectrum of impairment, ranging from mild worry to incapacitating withdrawal from social contact.
- Subtypes include generalized anxiety disorder, obsessive-compulsive disorder (OCD), school phobia, selective mutism, panic disorder, social anxiety, specific phobias.
- Estimated prevalence range up to 10%.

Separation/Anxiety and School Refusal

- Developmental separation anxiety should be outgrown by the school years. Persistent reluctance to leave an attachment figure with associated distress even in anticipation is indication of disorder. Comorbid depression possible in up to a third. Probable genetic contribution to etiology.

General Anxiety Disorder

- Child is consumed by worry over daily life stressors to the point of demonstrating panic sx, restlessness, somatic complaints, or insomnia.

Panic Disorder

- Sx: pounding heartbeat, dizziness, nausea, sweating triggered by ordinary events, usually outside the home. Avoidance behavior prevents normal school functioning and social contacts.

Selective Mutism

- Sx: failure to speak in specific social situations despite speaking in other situations. Children speak normally at home or when alone with parents, but otherwise fail to speak at school or elsewhere. Other sx: excessive shyness, withdrawal, dependency on parents, oppositional behavior. Mute children report that they want to speak in social settings but are afraid to do so.

Obsessive-Compulsive Disorder

- Obsessions are unwanted intrusive fixed or repetitive ideas, thoughts, images, or impulses; a compulsion is an irresistible impulse to act regardless of the irrationality of the motivation. Manifestations include body dysmorphic disorder, obsessions regarding germs and repetitive washing, ritualized counting, hoarding.
- Dx:
  - Confirmation via psychiatric referral. Complete H+P with screening labs to r/o physical etiology of sx complex and identify comorbidities (ADHD, Tourette, pediatric autoimmune neuropsychiatric disorders associated with streptococcus infections).
- Rx:
  - Cognitive-behavioral therapy for nonpharmacologic intervention. SSRIs; combination of psychosocial and pharmacologic rx for best outcome. Clomipramine as TCA alternative. Benzodiazepines only for short-term management of crises. For OCD, partial rather than complete remission is rx goal.

13.3 Depression

General Ref

- http://brightfutures.aap.org/3rd_Edition_Guidelines_and_Pocket_Guide.html
- *Contemp Pediatr* 2005;22:2, "Recognizing Bipolar Disorder"
- *N Engl J Med* 2002;347(9):667
- Osborne, *Pediatrics*, "Sadness and Depressive Disorders"

- *Pediatr Ann* 2007;36:9, "Pediatric Mood Disorders"
- *Pediatr Rev* 2009;30(6):199–205

Def

- DSM criteria similar as for adults but with pediatric clinical manifestations. One of "core sx" should be present:
  - Depressed or irritable mood most of the time, on most d
  - Loss of interest or pleasure in most activities

Epidem

- Estimated prevalence < 1% prepubertal, 1–3% peripubertal, 3–6% adolescence. Boys/girls equal prevalent in early childhood; 2:1 female in adolescence.
- Mean length of major depressive disorder (MDD) episode is 7–9 months; most recover by 2 yr.
- Relapse common: 70% within 5 yr.
- 10% depressed adolescents have suicidal ideation; suicide 3rd leading cause of death in teens.

Etiology

- Genetic contribution around 50% per twin and family studies.
- Physiologic basis may be variations in receptor function for serotonin neurotransmission.
- Environmental stressors may trigger an episode, unmasking genetic risk.
- Adverse childhood events and poor family functioning frequently complicate any treatment plan.
- Comorbid psychiatric diagnoses common: ADHD, anxiety, ODD, learning disorder (LD), eating disorders, substance abuse.

Dx

- Psychiatric referral and/or familiar screening tools (PHQ-9 available online).

- Address suicidal ideation; psychosocial hx to uncover triggers (abuse, substance abuse, other toxic exposures).
- Physical exam for physical etiology: hypo or hyperthyroidism, chronic inflammatory conditions, neurologic disorders, anemia. Labs rarely useful.

Rx

- Refer complex cases with multiple comorbid diagnoses, suicidal ideation, concerns about possible bipolar illness to psychiatrist.
- Family and pt education; suicide contract; remove firearms from home; combination psychotherapy + pharmacologic rx = best course. Cognitive behavioral therapy and interpersonal therapy effective; SSRIs most common: start low, titrate up slowly; transient gi side effects possible. Recommend SSRIs with longer half-life to decrease withdrawal sx effect if missed dose. Check pts in 1 wk. Caution pt re drug–drug interactions.

Bipolar Disorder

- Can present as depression with no prior hx of mania. Estimated 20% of childhood MDD evolves into bipolar disorder.
- Family hx increases risk. Sx complex: grandiosity, flight of ideas, decreased need for sleep.
- "Affective storms" describes rapid cycling of extreme temper tantrums (result in property damage) that only last hr.
- Euphoria might express itself as prolonged silliness, not age appropriate, but more commonly is persistent irritability, negativity, and anger.
- Aggressive behaviors, substance abuse, or unintentional recreational overdoses may lead to hospitalizations or incarceration.
- Rx includes mood stabilizers (lithium, anticonvulsants) and atypical antipsychotics (may require periodic metabolic screening—lipids, TSH, chemistry profile). Side effects include type 2 DM and tardive dyskinesia.

13.4 Tourette Syndrome

General Ref

- *Neurol Clin North Am* 1997;15:2
- *Contemp Pediatr* 2004;21:8
- http://www.tsa-usa.org/Medical/medsci.html
- *J Child Neurol* 2006;21(8), entire issue

Def

- Presence of multiple motor tics (and at least 1 vocal tic at some point), occurring daily for 1 yr, causing impairment in functioning (may have period of remission up to 3 months).
- "Chronic motor tics" have either motor or vocal stereotypic movements, but not both.
- "Transient tic disorder" lasts < 12 months. Coprolalia is a *rare* finding.

Epidem

- Three to four times as common in males. Tic intensity maximized at onset of puberty and then often wanes. Prevalence in childhood approx 4–10:10,000, declining to 0.5:10,000 in adults. Polygenic multifactorial inheritance likely; no current genetic test available; 10–15% risk in first-degree relatives, 70% concordance in identical twins.

Pathophys

- Unknown. Abnormalities in D2 receptors in caudate likely. Pts describe "premonitory urge": a sensory discomfort in the muscle group about to tic. The concept of an "urge relief cycle" posits that a motor urge leads to the tics; a cognitive urge leads to the OCD.

Dx

- No lab or genetic tests exist; based on clinical findings. Questionnaires help quantitate the tics and guide therapy (Y-GTSS "Yale Global Tic Severity Scale").

Sx

- Tics begin in early childhood as simple motor or phonic tics, become more complex over time. Most common: eye blinking, nose wrinkling, facial grimaces, shoulder or neck jerking. Complex tics can be hand gestures, repeated touching or smelling an object, lip licking, hair pulling, posturing. Phonic tics can range from sniffing to barking, coughing, clicking, repeating sounds, echolalia. Impulsive socially inappropriate language (disinhibition in criticizing body odor or looks of others) may be a type of tic.

Comorbidities

- ADHD, OCD, LD, affective disorder, mood disorders, sleep disorder, ODD are all common. ADHD present in 50% and is a common presenting complaint. Up to 25% have OCD severe enough to need interventions.

Rx

- Clonidine for sleep onset; Tenex has limited efficacy. Neuroleptics may decrease tics but side effects are obesity, sedation, and dyskinesia. Rx for comorbidities: stimulants for ADHD; SSRIs for anxiety or OCD.

13.5   Autism Spectrum Disorder

General Ref

- *Pediatrics* 2007;120(5):1162–1216
- *Pediatrics* 2009;123(5):1383–1386

Cause

- Biologically based. Characterized by qualitative differences in social interaction, language development, and self-regulation. Cause unknown, leading to inappropriate attribution to immunizations and thimerosal.

Epidem

- 6 per 1000 births in North American and Europe.
- Approximately one-third meet DSM criteria for autistic disorder; rest categorized as Asperger or pervasive developmental disorder not otherwise specified (PDD-NOS).
- 4:1 male.

Pathophys

- Can be "secondary" to certain genetic syndromes: Down, fragile X, tuberous sclerosis, neurofibromatosis type 1, phenylketonuria, fetal alcohol syndrome, Rett, Angelman, velo-cardio-facial.
- Linked to older parental age.
- Macrocephaly noted in 30%.
- Linked to fetal rubella, valproate exposure, thalidomide.
- Genetic interaction with "second hit" environmental trigger is leading hypothesis.
- Sibling recurrence rate 6%; monozygotic twin concordance shows 60% (90% for expanded definition).

Sx

- Commonly language delay, although not apparent until 18 months.
- Parents may note deficiencies in "joint attention" in infants; normal infants show enjoyment in sharing an object or experience with another person, look back and forth.
- Other sx might include resistance to cuddling, poor reciprocity.

Si

- Social skills deficits (lack of imitative behavior, lack of interaction with peers); language delay (absence of speech, monotone, echolalia, giant words; 25% may have regression of language in 2nd yr of life); quirky language (fixation on few topics, self-centered odd language), variations in play (repeated manipulation of wheels rather than use as toy car, lining up the crayons vs coloring, ignoring peers); stereotypies (flapping, rocking); excessive response to transitions (tantrums, self-injurious behavior); excessive attachment to special objects, rituals.

Comorbidities

- Association with MR lower as spectrum expands (now 25–30%). Rare savants.
- Seizures in 11–39%, although routine EEG not recommended.
- High frequency of gi disturbance (gas, vomiting, constipation, etc.) in about half.
- Sleep disorders.
- Psychiatric comorbidities include anxiety, OCD, ADHD, depression, aggression/explosive behaviors, self-injurious behaviors.

Dx

- AAP promotes use of formal screening tools at 18- and 24-month visit.
- If positive screens supported by clinical interview and observations, refer for hearing assessment and formal developmental evaluation.

Lab

- None to make dx.
- If MR also present, karyotype and fragile X testing generally done.
- If Rett considered, specific testing (MECP2).

- EEG if seizures suspected, metabolic workup if associated with odors or cyclic vomiting, imaging for tuberous sclerosis lesions if neurocutaneous findings, lead if pica, etc.

Rx

- Early intervention programs using "applied behavioral analysis" and other models.
- Social skills instruction, occupational therapy for self-help skills, and sensory integration are all of use.
- Older high-functioning children may be mainstreamed but need classroom modifications to process directions and promote appropriate social interactions.
- Medical management targets comorbidities. Sudden deteriorations of behavior often have environmental triggers that should be addressed before resorting to medications with potential toxicity. Approximately 40% of children with autism are on some psychotropic medication.
- Complementary and alternative medicine (CAM) approaches:
  - Used by up to 90% of parents.
  - Omega fatty acid supplements show promise; results inconclusive with gluten-restricted diets; likewise dairy restrictions.

13.6 Sleep Disorders

General Ref

- *Pepediatrics* 2003;111(5 Pt 1):e628–e635.
- *N Engl J Med* 2005;353:803–810, "Chronic Insomnia"
- *Pediatr Rev* 2006;27:455–462
- *Pediatr Rev* 1996;17:87–92

Def

- Insomnia includes difficulty falling asleep, sleep maintenance (night or early wakening), or quality of sleep (OSAS, parasomnias, movement disorders).

Norms for Sleep

- Infants usually sleep 13–15 hr per d; toddlers 11–12 hr; school-aged children 10–11 hr; teenagers 9 hr.
- At all ages, children and adults cycle through different sleep stages and have periodic arousals (approximately every 90 min). Wakenings that occur in the absence of the ability to self-soothe back down lead to sleep disruption.

Pathophys

- Insomnia induced by psychosocial stressors, caffeine use, alcohol and all drugs of abuse.
- Secondary insomnia from uncontrolled cough illness, chronic pain, hyperthyroidism, airway problems, restless legs, psychiatric conditions.
- Bedtime resistance and sleep-onset delay are associated with late TV watching, in particular with the TV in the bedroom.

Factors That Promote Sleep

- Dtime exercise; dark quiet room at comfortable temperature; regular schedule with minimal variation in time of waking, onset, and naps; no exciting TV; regular nighttime routine; same bed as for naps.
- Parent training to promote good "sleep hygiene" in infants and toddlers popularized by Ferber in 1990s: child to self-soothe back to sleep.

Delayed Sleep Phase Syndrome

- Extremely common in teens: result of sleeping late on wkends/holid then unable to return to normal sleep/wake schedule. Resolve by cutting back wake time in 15-min intervals daily or delay bedtime by few hr daily until desired schedule achieved.

Obstructive Sleep Apnea Syndrome

- Typically associated in children with huge tonsils and/or adenoids or palatal hypotonia.
- Hx of persistent "heroic" snoring with pauses, snorting, or choking; sweating with restless sleep is suggestive.
- Dtime fatigue, mood changes, poor concentration, and inattention are blamed on obstruction.
- Tonsillectomy and adenoidectomy resolves 80–90% of the cases, with the remainder requiring bilevel positive airway pressure and/or weight loss.

Movement Disorders of Sleep

- 2% of children meet criteria for restless leg syndrome (RLS) or periodic limb movement disorder (PLMD).
- Children with RLS report an urge to move that is usually associated with unpleasant sensations, sx that are worse at rest, relieved by movement, and most severe at night.
- PLMD presents with more stereotypic repetitive muscle movements resembling myoclonic jerks that can wake the child, leading to dtime sleepiness.
- Medical rx for both disorders is unsatisfactory, although occasionally iron supplementation can decrease sx of RLS.

Medications for Sleep

- 2–3% of pediatric visits in one survey involved sleep issues.
- 75% of practitioners recommended OTC medications, typically antihistamine or melatonin (valerian root or chamomile tea for natural rx), and 50% prescription medication.
- Special needs children with MR, autism, and ADHD were most common group getting prescription, and clonidine the most popular medication.
- Melatonin dose: 3 mg given 30 min before sleep; clonidine dose half of 0.1 mg tab, increasing if needed.

- Both trazodone and mirtazapine are frequently used, with starting doses of 25 and 7.5 mg, respectively, with the former rarely causing priapism in teen males.
- *None* of these medications are effective in maintaining sleep once their sedative effect has worn off, and none have been studied well for pediatric use.

Chapter 14

Dermatology

14.1 Eczema

General Ref

- *J Allergy Clin Immunol* 2003;112:S118–127
- *Br J Dermatol* 2008;158:754–765

Cause

- Disease of childhood, often associated with family hx of atopy

Epidem

- Prevalence 12–20%.
- Onset 1st yr of life.
- Uncommon < 2 months of age.
- 50% may develop asthma or hay fever.
- 50% resolved by 12 yr of age.
- 75% resolved by 16 yr of age.

Pathophys

- Ref: *Trends Mol Med* 2008;14:20–27, *J Allergy Clin Immunol* 2007;120:1406–1412.
- Recent studies have shown that the protein filaggrin plays a key role in providing a skin barrier against the environment. Mutations on the profilaggrin gene *FLG* causing loss of function are present in 10% of the population and have been

found to be a major risk factor for the development of eczema (atopic dermatitis).

S+S

- Itching main symptom at all ages; skin becomes excoriated, erythematous with crusting and weeping from scratching and rubbing; may result in thickening of the skin.

Course

- Breastfeeding protective; delays onset but does not alter natural hx

Complications

- Secondary infection with staphylococcus or streptococcus. Herpes virus can spread rapidly in atopic skin (eczema herpeticum).

Lab

- Clinical dx:
  - May have elevated IgE levels.
  - If severe or atypical in presentation, consider excluding an immunodeficiency disorder.

Rx

- Emollients mainstay of treatment. Ointments preferred to creams; apply liberally several times a d.
- Topical steroids: use with care during acute exacerbations; 1% hydrocortisone ointment twice daily; avoid use on the face.
- Topical tacrolimus or pimecrolimus (Elidel) for children > 2 yr; short-term use may reduce need for topical steroids.
- Oral antihistamine for itching.
- Antibiotics and antivirals if secondary infection.

14.2 Viral Exanthems

General Ref:

- *Pediatr Infect Dis J* 2009;28:250
- *Pediatr Infect Dis J* 2008;27:533
- *N Engl J Med* 2005;352:768

Cause

- An acute viral syndrome; all viruses can cause an exanthem (if mucosa also involved called an enanthem).

Epidem

- Common; exact incidence unknown. In the United States, enteroviral and adenoviral exanthems are the most common.

S+S

- May be difficult to differentiate from drug eruptions, rickettsial infections, and allergic reactions.
- May classify according to the type of rash:
  - Morbilliform (morbilli: measles-like): most common. Discrete maculopapular pink to red macules. Includes adenovirus, parvovirus B19, measles, enterovirus.
  - Epstein-Barr virus (EBV): roseola, erythema infectiosum, rubella, dengue, mumps, cytomegalovirus, respiratory syncytial virus, echovirus.
  - Papular acrodermatitis (Gianotti-Crosti syndrome): distinct entity seen with cytomegalovirus, hepatitis B, coxsackie A16, and EBV. Acral distribution of large flat-topped erythematous papules. Lesions are not pruritic; commonly affect elbows, knees, buttocks, and cheeks; rash may precede upper respiratory tract sx; 85% < 3 yr; may affect school-age children. Rash persists for 2–8 wk and may recur.

- Vesiculobullous eruptions: include herpes simplex virus, varicella virus, coxsackie A16 (hand foot and mouth disease), echovirus, influenza virus.

Course

- Usually self-limiting and benign in healthy children. Immunosuppressed children at high risk of complications.

Complications

- Secondary bacterial infections, viral meningitis, or encephalitis that may result in neurologic sequelae

Rx

- Morbilliform: no specific treatment; supportive care (i.e., fluid, antipyretics).
- Measles: children $\geq$ 1 yr given single dose of vitamin A 200,000 IU; 6–12 months of age, give 100,000 IU.
- Papular acrodermatitis: no specific treatment; counsel re prolonged course.
- Vesiculobullous: herpes simplex virus: oral acyclovir 20–40 mg/kg per d safe and effective in children if initiated within 72 hr. Valacyclovir or famciclovir are alternatives. Chickenpox: treatment is supportive. Secondary bacterial infections most common complication and should be treated with po antistaphylococcus drug (e.g., dicloxacillin). Hand, foot, and mouth disease: supportive treatment.
- Prevent disease through immunization.
- Immunocompromised children with severe entero or parvovirus infection may benefit from IVIG.
- Parvovirus may cause an aplastic crisis requiring blood transfusion.

14.3 Acne

General Ref

- *Dermatol Clin* 2009;27:33–42
- *Cutis* 2006;78:5–11

Cause

- Hypertrophic sebaceous glands lead to increased sebum production. *Propionibacterium acnes* is the bacteria involved.

Epidem

- Most common during teen yr

Pathophys

- Hyperkeratinization or plugging of follicles.
- *P. acnes* proliferation is critical to the development of the inflammatory lesion and causes the production of chemotactic factors.
- A relative androgen excess may lead to increased sebum production.

S+S

- Papules on an erythematous base; pustules and comedones

Rx

- Mild:
  - Benzoyl peroxide: a keratolytic that decreases *P. acnes*
  - Tretinoins: mainstay of topical acne treatment (e.g., Retin-A)
  - Azelaic acid bacteriostatic against *P. acnes*: useful monotherapy alternative to retinoids
  - Tazarotene: third-generation retinoid for mild to moderate acne

- Moderate:
  - Oral contraceptives
  - Tetracycline 250–500 mg twice daily or doxycycline 100 mg daily until lesions resolved
  - Alternatives: clindamycin or erythromycin
- Severe cystic acne:
  - Retinoids: isotretinoin 1–4 mg/kg po every d for 4 months; should consult dermatology

14.4 Kawasaki Disease (Mucocutaneous Lymph Node Syndrome)

General Ref

- *Lancet* 2004;364(9433):533–544
- *Arch Pediatr Adolesc Med* 2004;158(12):1166–1169

Cause

- Unknown; a small and medium vessel vasculitis

Epidem

- 6 months to 4 yrs of age; peak at end of 1st yr; leading cause of acquired heart disease in children in United States

Pathophys

- Clinical and immunologic similarities to staphylococcus and streptococcus toxic shock syndromes have led to suggestions of a bacterial toxin acting as a superantigen.

S+S

- Diagnostic criteria:
  - Fever > 5 d with 4 or more of the following:
    - Nonexudative conjunctival injection

- Mucous membranes involvement of upper respiratory tract: fissured lips, strawberry tongue, exudative pharyngitis
- Cervical lymphadenopathy
- Polymorphous rash
- Edema or erythema of hands and feet or peeling of fingers and toes
- Other findings: aseptic meningitis with child very irritable; arthralgia common; uveitis in up to 80% of cases

Course

- Typically self-limited with resolution within 12 d without treatment

Complications

- Coronary artery aneurysm; cardiomyopathy

Lab

- CBC + differential; elevated WCC with a left shift, mild anemia, platelets low normal or high early with thrombocytosis by 2nd week
- ESR elevated; often > 100 mm
- EKG: acute phase: prolonged PR interval, decreased QRS voltage, flattened T waves, ST changes

Xray

- Chest Xray: may show an enlarged heart
- Echocardiogram: aneurysm usually noted by 3–4 wk; may be seen as early as 6 d

Rx

- Bed rest until afebrile > 72 hr: avoid strenuous activity even if asymptomatic due to risk of myocardial involvement during acute phase.

- IVIG 2g/kg 1 dose over 10 hr; repeat if no response or if recrudescence of sx (failure to respond to IVIG associated with increased risk of coronary artery aneurysm).
- High-dose aspirin 80–100 mg/kg per d; divided doses for 14 d or until afebrile for 48 hr; then decrease to 3–5 mg/kg per d until platelet count and ESR return to normal.
- High-dose methylprednisone (30 mg/kg per d; once a d for 1–3 d) has been used with benefit in children who fail to respond to IVIG (*J Pediatr* 1996;128(1):146–149, *Pediatr Int* 2001;43(3):211–217).
- Live vaccines should be postponed for 11 months in children who receive IVIG.

14.5   Diaper Dermatitis

General Ref

- *Arch Pediatr Adolesc Med* 2000;154:943–946
- *Curr Med Res Opin* 2004;20:645–649

Cause

- Irritant, infantile seborrheic dermatitis, candida infection, atopic eczema
- Less common causes: acrodermatitis enteropathica, Langerhans cell histiocytosis, Wiskott-Aldrich syndrome

S+S

- Irritant contact dermatitis:
  - Most common cause: irritant effect of urine and or feces on the skin
  - May occur if diapers are not changed frequently enough, poorly absorbent diapers, or if infant has diarrhea
  - Rash erythematous, scalded appearance, characteristically sparing the flexures and affecting the perineal region, convexities of the buttocks, and lower abdomen

- Rx: frequent diaper changes, topical emollients first-line therapy (e.g., zinc oxide, Vaseline petrolatum, Desitin, Balmex, Triple Paste)
- Candida diaper dermatitis:
  - Erythematous rash that includes the skin flexures with associated satellite lesions.
  - Rx: topical antifungal cream (e.g., nystatin, clotrimazole, miconazole). Apply 3 times per d beneath the barrier cream until resolved.
- Infantile seborrheic dermatitis:
  - Involvement of the diaper area with a scaly erythematous rash that includes the flexures
  - Similar rash on scalp; may involve flexure surfaces, face
  - Rx: low potency topical corticosteroid cream twice daily for a maximum of 7 d
- Atopic eczema:
  - Diaper area usually spared due to moist environment; if a rash does occur, will be itchy with signs of scratching and the typical atopic rash on the rest of the body
  - Rx: low potency corticosteroid 2–3 times daily; maximum 7 d
- Langerhans cell histiocytosis:
  - May present with severe recalcitrant red or brown scaly papules, petechiae, or erosions in the diaper area, scalp, and intertriginous zones

14.6 Pityriasis Rosea

General Ref

- *J Am Acad Dermatol* 2006;54:82–85
- *Cochrane Database Syst Rev* 2007;(2):CD005068

Cause

- Common self-limiting disorder thought to be viral in origin

Epidem

- Occurs in 10–35 yr age group

Pathophys

- Papulosquamous disorder affecting trunk and limbs

S+S

- Usually begins with single oval scaly macule, the herald patch, followed in a few ds by smaller macules on the trunk (in a "Christmas tree distribution") on the upper arms and thighs. May be itchy.

Course

- Resolves spontaneously in 4–6 wk

Lab

- Skin scrapings to r/o *Tinea versicolor* or dermatophytes

Rx

- Usually resolves spontaneously after 6 wk; commonly asymptomatic; provide reassurance.
- First line:
  - Topical corticosteroids suppress inflammatory component of disease.
  - Emollients may help.
  - Oral antihistamines for itch.
- Second line:
  - Ultraviolet b
- Third line:
  - Extensive eruptions: oral prednisone may help.
  - Oral erythromycin 25–40 mg/kg divided doses produces complete clearance after 2 wk in most pts.

14.7 Urticaria

General Ref

- *N Engl J Med* 2002;346:175
- *Curr Allergy Asthma Rep* 2008;8:278–287

Cause

- Several mechanisms produce urticaria:
  - Allergic type 1 hypersensitivity reaction (drugs, foods). IgE activates mast cells, which then produce histamine and other immune mediators, causing urticaria and itching.
  - Hypersensitivity reaction type II with activated complement products (C3a, C5a), causing mast cell activation.
  - Type I or III hypersensitivity reaction; increased vascular permeability activates the plasma kinin forming pathway. Increased kinins further increase vascular permeability, causing tissue edema and urticaria.
  - Nonimmunologic activation of mast cells. Opioids, some antibiotics may directly stimulate mast cells.

Epidem

- Affects 15–25% of general population; common in infancy and childhood, but incidence unknown; some studies suggest 3% in preschoolers and 2% in older children. Increased incidence in children with atopic dermatitis.

Pathophys

- Dilation of small venules and capillaries in the superficial dermis. Plasma leakage and short lived; itchy raised wheals due to dermal edema.

DERMATOLOGY

S+S

- Raised, itchy erythematous wheals; target lesions of erythema multiforme

Course

- Resolves spontaneously in most cases, persistence for > 6 wk described as chronic urticaria.

Lab

- Clinical dx

Rx

- Systemic or oral H1 receptor antagonist antihistamines (e.g., loratadine)
- Doxepin useful in chronic urticaria

14.8 Scabies

General Ref

- *Postgrad Med J* 2005;81:7–11
- *Lancet* 2006;367:1767–1774

Cause

- Scabies is a parasitic infestation of the skin caused by the arthropod *Sarcoptes scabiei*.

Epidem

- Worldwide distribution; more prevalent in developing countries

Pathophys

- A delayed-type IV hypersensitivity reaction to the mites, ova, and feces under the skin. Causes sx within 4–6 wk after the initial infection. Transmission requires human contact.

S+S

- An acute pruritic dermatitis with erythematous papules, excoriation, crusts, and pustules.
- Pruritus intense and often worse at night.
- Children may have any part of skin involved; infants have hundreds of lesions; older children and adults have few.
- Burrows pathognomonic.

Course

- Itching may persist 7–10 d after successful treatment, but there should be no new lesions.

Complications

- Norwegian scabies (diffuse hyperkeratosis, crusting and lichenification of skin in children who cannot scratch effectively), secondary impetigo.

Lab

- Scraping unscratched burrow and examining under oil immersion: female mite and eggs seen

Rx

- Application of a scabicide:
  - Permethrin 5% approved first-line treatment from > 2 months of age by the CDC; applied from chin to toes and for a period of 10–12 hr, after which it should be washed off. The treatment is repeated in 1 wk.
  - Lindane; reports of resistance in the United States.
  - Malathion.
  - Ivermectin 200 µg/kg single dose for refractory cases or those who cannot tolerate topical treatment.
  - Antihistamines and topical antibiotics may be used for itching and to treat any secondary infection.

14.9   Tinea

General Ref

- *Cochrane Database Syst Rev* 2007;(3):CD001434
- *Pediatr Dermatol* 2001;18:465–468

Cause

- *Tinea capitis: Microsporum canis*: human-to-human transmission does not occur; humans terminal host (found in cats, dogs, and rodents).
- *Trichophyton tonsurans*: human-to-human infection occurs: sharing hats, scarves, combs, etc.
  - *T. corporis: M. canis, T. tonsurans, T. verrucosum, T. mentagrophytes*
  - *T. pedis* (athlete's foot: *T. rubrum* and *T. mentagrophytes* most common)

Epidem

- Common; associated with overcrowding, hot and humid climates; *T. pedis* more common in adolescents; *T. cruris* unusual before adolescence

Pathophys

- Dermatophytes are fungal infections that invade and proliferate on the outer layer of the epidermis, hair, and nails.

S+S

- *T. capitis*: characteristic noninflammatory stage lasting 2–8 wk, followed by an inflammatory phase with hair loss. Enlarged suboccipital or postcervical lymph nodes.
- *T. corporis*: typical annular to circular erythematous, scaly raised border with central clearing. Lesions may be multiple. Epidemics may occur in wrestlers (*T. gladiatorum*). If misdiagnosed and treated with steroids, border may be lost (*T. incognito*).

- *T. pedis:* annular erythema with vesicles and erosions on the instep, fissuring between the toes.
- *T. cruris:* erythematous scaly rash in inguinal area and inner thighs.

Complications
- Scarring may result in permanent hair loss.

Lab
- *T. capitis:* Wood's light examination (hairs fluoresce yellow-green), KOH examination, fungal culture
- *T. corporis:* KOH scrapings from border of lesions; culture not usually needed
- *T. pedis:* KOH fungal scrapings, fungal culture
- *T. cruris:* KOH exam of scrapings from border

Rx
- *T. capitis:* griseofulvin 20 mg/kg per d po for 4 wk, often need to treat for 2–3 months; terbinafine 3 mg/kg per d po for 2–4 wk. Treat affected animals.
- Fungal infections not involving hair or nails: topical antifungals may be used applied twice daily as cream or solution (e.g., terbinafine, ketoconazole, nystatin).

14.10   Alopecia Areata

General Ref
- *Pediatr Dermatol* 2002;19:298

Cause
- Chronic inflammatory process of hair follicles and nails

Epidem
- Most common cause of hair loss in children

Pathophys
- Autoimmune, T-lymphocyte mediated

S+S

- Patchy hair loss in otherwise normal skin; in most cases one or more coin-sized lesions; total hair loss from scalp alopecia totalis does occur.

Course

- Nonscarring hair loss; spontaneous resolution in > 95% after weeks to months; prognosis more guarded in children with atopic disorders.

Rx

- Most resolve spontaneously; no treatment alters long-term prognosis:
  - Intralesional corticosteroids
  - Topical immunotherapy
  - Topical corticosteroids
  - Anthralin (dithranol)
  - Topical minoxidil
  - Phototherapy

14.11   Other Causes of Hair Loss

- Behavioral: traumatic hair pulling, following burns
- Scalp atrophy: lichen planus, systemic lupus
- Following infection: *T. capitis*

14.12   Malignant Melanoma

General Ref

- *Int J Dermatol* 2005;44:715–723
- *Int J Cancer* 2007;120:1116–1122

Cause

- Risk factors: sun exposure, tanning beds (*Cancer Epidemiol Biomarkers Prev* 2005;14:562–526). PUVA therapy used in the treatment of psoriasis and other skin conditions (*J Am Acad Dermatol* 2001;44:755–761)

Epidem

- Rare in childhood; uncommon but increased frequency in adolescents

S+S

- Ref: Weston, Lane, and Morelli, *Colour Textbook of Pediatric Dermatology*

Lab

- Pathology

Rx

- Surgical excision and bx rx of choice with yearly follow-up and surveillance.
- Counsel re recognizing change in lesions, protection from the sun, importance of regular follow-up.

Table 14.1   ABCDs of Melanoma Detection

Asymmetry: lesion with an irregular shape

Border: uneven, notched, or irregular

Color: areas of red, white, and/or blue within a brown area

Diameter: > 10 mm

Evolution: rapid change in any of above over weeks is concerning

---

DERMATOLOGY

14.13   Head Lice

General Ref

- AAP guideline, 2003;110(3):638–643

Cause

- *Pediculosis capitis* infestation. Adult louse is gray, size of sesame seed. Eggs (nits) incubate near scalp due to body heat of host; hatch in 10–14 d. Viable nits match hair color, whereas empty casings are whitish. Adhere strongly to hair. Live louse unlikely to survive > 48 hr away from host.

Epidem

- 6–12 million cases per yr; most common in children. Not linked to disease or uncleanliness.

S+S

- Scalp itch.
- Live lice or nits close to scalp. Wet comb and empty on white towel for accuracy.

Complications

- Social ostracism, community anxiety. AAP is against NO NIT policies, although nit removal helpful in decreasing dx confusion and retreatment.

Rx

- Chemical pediculicide: OTC products containing permethrin 1%. Can consider prescription form (5%) if resistance suspected. Pyrethrin OTC products may also be effective. Resistance traced to point mutations in sodium channel genes of organisms (*Arch Dermatol* 2003:139:994). Ovide (Malathion) is most ovicidal but flammable.

- Limited data suggest adding TMP-SMX to chemical rx increases success rates. Antibiotic kills commensal flora in louse gi tract. Downside is antibiotic exposure, risk of systemic reactions:
- Nonchemical rx: occlusive measures include Nuvo shrink-wrapping technique: Massage Cetaphil lotion into hair, wait 2 min, comb out with fine-toothed comb (metal Lice Meister best), then dry with blow dryer. Can repeat wkly for 3 treatments to be careful. More than 95% cure rates (*Pediatrics* 2004;114[3]:e275–279; www.nuvoforheadlice.com).
- Wash recently used clothing, bath and bed linens; vacuum furniture, car seats; hats and other items can be put in plastic bags for 3 wk.

DERMATOLOGY

Chapter 15
General Topics

15.1   Abuse

General Ref

- *Pediatr Rev* 2004;25;264–277
- *Pediatrics* 2009;123(5):1430–1435
- AAP, *Diagnostic Imaging of Child Abuse*, section on radiology
- *Pediatrics* 2002;110:985

Def

- Child physical abuse: patterns of injury inflicted on child by caregiver, adult, older sibling, etc.

History

- Key finding is unexplained injury: hx inconsistent with findings or developmental stage of child.
  - Serial alterations in the hx to different questioners is common.
  - Concerning behaviors: recurrent injuries with a pattern of increasing severity; delay in seeking care; pattern of use of different medical facilities.
  - More common in homes with domestic violence, poverty, previous abuse of a sibling, hx of parents being abused as children.

Epidem

- Rates of overall child abuse/neglect approximately 12 in 1000.
- Physical abuse approximately 18% of cases (others = neglect, sexual abuse, emotional abuse).
- 1400 deaths per yr, of which 40% < 1 yr and 80% < 4 yr.
- Rates of abuse in the context of domestic violence estimated to be 30–60%.
- Long-term mental health issues in victims is public health concern.

Physical Exam

- Classic signs: bruises patterned into handprints or objects; bite marks; ligature mark/pinch marks; burns.
- Unclothed examination of the entire skin surface is necessary.
- Careful palpation of the skull and scalp for edema or step-offs.
- Oral exam looking for bruising and frenula tears from forced feeding.
- Retinal exam for hemorrhages.
- Chest bruising (in an infant) should trigger careful examination of the lungs and imaging for rib fractures, pneumothorax.
- Abdominal bruising is correlated with significant intra-abdominal injuries: hepatic or splenic rupture, intestinal hematomas or rupture.

Xray

- Pediatric emergency department should have skeletal survey protocol that includes AP of arms/forearms/thighs/legs. Hands posteroanterior (PA); feet PA or AP. Frontal and lateral skull, AP and lateral cervical spine, lateral lumbosacral (LS) spine, AP of abd/LS spine/pelvis, AP and lateral thorax (include thoracic spine and ribs). Oblique views of ribs if suspicion of rib fractures that doesn't show on standard view.

- Bone scan to supplement Xrays, but skeletal survey is mandatory < 2 yr.
- If clinical findings point to a skeletal injury not well delineated on films, orthopedic consultation and consideration of advanced modalities (MRI) is indicated.
- In the presence of radiographic injuries, radiologists should comment on general bone structure to defuse any future arguments regarding "brittle bones" (osteogenesis imperfecta or epiphyseal dysplasias).
- Head trauma:
  - CT without contrast is rapid and sensitive for acute blood collections that might require immediate intervention.
  - MRI takes sedation and may not be appropriate acutely, but it has the greatest yield for documenting intracranial injury after the acute phase (5–7 d). If MRI, include cervical spine.
- Chest/abdominal injuries:
  - CT is modality of choice.
  - Can delineate pulmonary contusions.
  - IV contrast is needed for delineating organ injury, but po contrast unnecessary.
- Shaken baby syndrome:
  - Sudden acceleration/deceleration from shaking.
  - Can present with vomiting and lethargy, "septic"-like behavior easy to mistake for meningitis. LP showing blood misinterpreted as traumatic tap.
  - Areas of hypoxic ischemic encephalopathy can later atrophy; CT should delineate acute changes related to subdural bleeding from torn bridging veins.
  - Chronic subdurals and intraparenchymal shearing lesions may only be detectable by MRI.
  - Ophthalmologic exam for hemorrhages indicated if suspected.

Lab

- Indicated by clinical factors; check international normalized ratio and PTT to document normal coagulation function.

Munchausen by Proxy

- Manufactured sx by caregiver. Most common sx: bleeding, apnea, altered mental status, diarrhea, emesis, skin rashes, FTT, or fever.
- Caregiver may report factitious events only witnessed by caretaker (seizure, apnea), feign disease states (heating the thermometer, putting blood in a body fluid), or induce disease (ipecac, laxatives, injecting saliva, irritating skin, giving drugs).
- Disappearance of sx when the child and caretaker are separated is diagnostic.

15.2   The Limping Child

General Ref

- *J Bone Joint Surg [Br]* 1999;81B:1029–1034
- *Pediatr Rev* 1995;16:458–465
- *Pediatr Rev* 2006;27;170–180
- Stotts, "Disorders of the hip" in Osborne *Pediatrics*, pp. 374–378

Def

- Alteration of gait due to discomfort.
- Must sort serious from benign etiology.

Diff Dx

- Possible etiologies: infectious, traumatic, rheumatologic, hematologic, structural, somaticization.

- Anatomic location may be in long bones, joints, or, rarely, the spine.
- Diff dx must factor pt age, presence/absence of fever, acuteness of onset.
- Hip most challenging site because is not visible or palpable.

Epidem

- ER study from United Kingdom showed 40% with hip synovitis; 30% no dx; 2% Perthes, 2% osteo, 15% soft tissue injury or toddler's fracture.
- Toxic synovitis most common dx in children 3–8 yr. Presents with antalgic gait or refusal to bear weight, often on awakening; low-grade fever, mild elevation of acute phase reactants (ESR in 30s); challenging to distinguish from early septic arthritis or osteoarthritis.
- Abnormal lab values, higher fever, discomfort on exam = likelihood of bacterial process.
- Discomfort to hip rotation: likely toxic synovitis; exquisite pain: likely septic joint.
- Xray to r/o trauma, anatomic abnormalities.
- Repeated episodes raise possibility of Legg-Perthes.
- Septic arthritis: medical emergency; requires surgical drainage, antibiotics.
- Toxic synovitis: self-resolution 3–7 d; symptomatic rx NSAIDs and rest.
- Rheumatologic conditions: juvenile idiopathic arthritis (JIA), acute rheumatic fever, Lyme disease, reactive arthritides, viral associated arthritis, lupus, Henoch-Schönlein purpura (HSP): all unusual in hip. HSP can present with enthesopathy prior to characteristic rash.
- Hematologic conditions: leukemia, sickle cell disease.
- Other possible etiologies: deep venous thrombosis, cancer (Ewing's, osteogenic sarcoma)
- Anatomic abnormalities: leg length discrepancies: abnormal gait, no acute pain. Secondary to developmental dislocation of

hip (careful hip exam for asymmetry or limited abduction for dx) or Legg-Perthes (typically in 4- to 8-yr-old active boy); subacute onset of limp; pain referred to knee, groin, thigh; Xrays to show subtle lucency under joint surface, which can progress to fragmentation and collapse of femoral head.

- Slipped capital femoral epiphysis (SCFE) occurs in early phases of puberty, thought to be due to a weak period for active growth plate. More common in males, African Americans; comorbidity of obesity; associated with hypothyroidism (check TSH in pts < 10 yr of age). May have acute presentation or subacute with gradual onset of discomfort (can be referred pain to knee or groin). Bilateral Xrays for comparison (r/o bilateral slip; subtle alterations in growth plate). Rx: crutches, no weight bearing. Screws to stabilize hip until close of growth plate.

15.3 Lipid Screening

General Ref

- *Pediatrics* 2008;122;198–208
- Ferranti and Newburger, *Up to Date*, October 2008

Def

- Preventive cardiology to r/o early atherosclerosis; pediatric interventions to prevent premature morbidity and mortality in adults.
- Obesity, hypertension, DM 1 and 2, past Kawasaki disease, tobacco addiction, atypical antipsychotics can accelerate genetic risk.
- Homozygosity for some familial lipid disorders leading to pediatric cardiovascular events is rare but possible.

Epidem

- Population studies show 70% or more of top 10th percentile with elevated lipids in childhood develop cholesterol levels > 200.
- Early intervention with lifestyle modification to prevent long-term complications.

Lab

- Childhood dyslipidemia (TC > 200, LDL-C > 130, HDL-C < 40–45, TG > 150 for teen or 130 for preteen). Current recommendation: screen children/adolescents with pos family hx of dyslipidemia or premature CVD if family hx unknown. If other CVD risk factors (overweight, hypertension, cigarette smoking, DM) present, use fasting lipid profile between ages 2–10 yr.
- Check lipids of children on atypical antipsychotics before initiation, re-check for 3–4 months; monitor annually.
- General recommendations for children:
  - Experts recommend all children > 2 yr receive < 30% of their calories as fat (saturated fat < 10% of calories). Total daily cholesterol target is < 200 mg. New AAP recommendation 1.5% milk for toddlers. Standard measures: eliminate trans-fats, restrict concentrated sweets (soda), eat balanced diet (fruits, vegetables, whole grains). Weight control/regular exercise. If child dx dyslipidemia, saturated fat reduction down to 7% of calories. Refer family to dietician.
- Nonpharmacologic intervention:
  - Increase exercise to elevate HDL-C (20 min, 3 times a wk; moderate exertion); dietary restrictions; supplemental fish oil, dietary fiber. No cigarette smoking or second-hand exposure.

- Medication management:
  - Not recommended for children < 8 yr.
  - Criteria for initiating meds (statins) include start of puberty and failure of 6–12 months of lifestyle modification to lower lipid levels.
  - In absence of other risk factors, lab cutoff value for meds is LDL-C > 190 with a treatment goal of 160.
  - Lower goal is recommended (110–130) if there is a family hx of early CVD or any 2 additional risk factors (BMI > 85th percentile, high BP, metabolic syndrome) or even 100 in presence of DM.
  - Past hx Kawasaki disease with aneurysms, chronic kidney disease, chronic inflammatory illness, cancer survivorship: All increase risk of future CVD and justify a more aggressive approach.

15.4   Ingestion

General Ref

- *Pediatr Rev* 2004;25;370–371
- Lange, *Poisoning and Drug Overdose*, 5th ed., 2007
- APLS *Pediatric Emergency Medicine Resource*, 4th ed., Chapter 8
- *Pediatr Rev* 2009:30:295–300

Def

- Consider toxic exposure if child presents with unexplained neurologic depression or irritability/seizures, vomiting/diarrhea, meiosis/mydriasis/nystagmus, respiratory depression, metabolic acidosis.
- Unusual odors may be sign; high index of suspicion, careful hx of potential toxins in the environment.

Epidem

- Pediatric ingestions = approximately half of 2.4 million annual calls to poison control centers.
- Leading causes of death are analgesics, sedatives, antipsychotics, and tricyclics.
- Adult relatives' or siblings' prescriptions that are mishandled are typically the source in young children and suicide gestures in teens.

Physical Exam

- ABCDE assessment, monitors and oxygen if indicated; documentation of mental status.
- Look for toxidrome (pupils, saliva, HR, BP, skin texture).
- Advanced airway management if severe impairment of mental status.

Lab

- CBC, chem.-20, INR, specific drug level(s), toxicology screen, EKG, chest Xray, depending on suspected toxin. Calculation of the anion gap done by $Na -(Cl + CO2) \rightarrow$ normal is 8–12. Calculation of osmolar gap $\rightarrow$ measured osmoles $-(2\,Na + glucose/18 + BUN/2.8 + ethanol/4)$.

General Management

- Call local poison control center for assistance; ipecac no longer recommended; gastric lavage controversial. Consider immediate dose of activated charcoal: 1–2 g/kg in young children; adult dose 50–100 g. First dose typically given in sorbitol to avoid complication of constipation, bezoar. For selected toxins (drugs with enterohepatic circulation) repeat doses given: continuous NG at 0.2 g/kg per hr, or approximately one-quarter dose every 1–4 hr (without cathartic; typical adult rate is 12.5/hr). Charcoal not useful for iron, lithium, hydrocarbons/solvents, caustics, alcohols, pesticides.

- Also decrease absorption via whole bowel irrigation with GoLYTELY: 500 mL/hr for toddlers, with adult dose 1–2 L/hr (goal: clear stools).
- Urinary alkalinization to enhance excretion: begin with 1 mEq/kg bolus, followed by IV solution of D5 "normal bicarbonate": add 150 mEq bicarb to liter of D5. If no renal failure, add 20–40 KCl per liter to the fluid. Infuse at generous maintenance rate.
- Refer to tertiary center for hemodialysis: life-threatening methanol, ethylene glycol, ASA, phenobarbital, lithium, theophylline.

Antidotes

- Available for specific toxins once identified; contact local poison control.
- NAC for acetaminophen, flumazenil for benzodiazepines, and naloxone for opiates. FAB for digoxin, physostigmine for anticholinergics, atropine for anticholinesterases.
- Chelating agents for lead and other metals, deferoxamine for iron, ethanol or fomepizole for antifreeze, and methylene blue use for methemoglobinemia.
- Acetaminophen: now an IV as well as po. IV has shorter duration. Whether or not treatment needed based on Rumack nomogram with level drawn 4 hr after time of ingestion.
  - Opioids: CNS depression, pinpoint pupils with complication of depressed respirations. May need to specify on toxic screen for buprenorphine. Naloxone 0.1 mg/kg or 2–4 mg in older child; repeat bolus or set up drip.
  - Clonidine: acts like opioid, small pupils. Bradycardia and hypotension common, although immediately *after* the ingestion can be hypertensive. Use of naloxone controversial and potentially dangerous. Management includes

continuous monitoring, respiratory support, fluids to support BP, and, rarely, inotropes.

Foreign Body Ingestions

- Coins likely catch in either cricopharyngeal junction or distal esophagus; if pass into stomach, will generally exit the GI tract without difficulty.
- Persistent drooling or dysphagia suggests need for endoscopic removal. Either radiography or metal detector can localize. Special concerns arise with sharp objects: pins or nails > 4–6 cm tend to have difficulty making the corners through the small bowel; best to remove them from the stomach.
- Button batteries are of concern. Can leak caustic chemicals or cause erosions by setting up an electric current. Esophageal batteries should be removed; if in the stomach, should document passage.
- Magnets can attract when more than one ingested and lead to bowel wall necrosis; case reports include sepsis and death as complications. May be hard to tell more than one on Xray. Compass on abdominal wall may be attracted. Surgical consultation advisable.

15.5   Lead Poisoning

General Ref

- *N Engl J Med* 2003;348(16):1517–1525
- *N Engl J Med* 1983;309:1089–1093
- *Pediatr Rev* 2000;21:327–335

Def

- Lead is childhood toxin. Recent data suggest there is no threshold below which lead exposure is "safe"; there are subtle but measurable effects on cognition at levels 1–10, with estimated IQ drop of 7.4 across that range.

Pathophys

- Lead is a divalent cation (Pb^{++}) that incorporates itself into enzyme systems throughout the body. In the bone marrow, disruption of the synthetic pathway for hgb leads to basophilic stippling of the rbcs; generally *only* in what are now considered very high levels (> 25). Interference with calcium deposition at high levels can lead to characteristic "lead lines" on Xrays of long bones. Long-term renal toxicity from low levels is suspected, with both glomerular and tubular function affected (occupational exposures in adults).
- Predominant concern is developmental impairment from CNS toxicity.
- At low levels, effects are nonspecific and act in concert with poverty, social dysfunction, and poor nutrition.

Dx

- Screen at-risk children at age 1 and 2.
- Risk factors include living in older housing (pre-1960), spending time in older housing (especially if chipping paint or renovation), having a sibling or playmate with elevated level.
- Imported toys, lead glazed pottery use, and use of tainted imported pharmaceuticals or herbs have been linked to toxicity.
- Severe exposures can lead to sx; consider environmental hx and lead level in, for example, an immigrant child with unexplained neurologic or gi symptoms.

Prevention

- Public health efforts toward prevention have led to lower levels.

Rx

- There are no medical interventions recommended for the vast majority of children with elevation of blood lead level (EBLL). Adequate dietary iron and calcium intake is thought to competitively decrease lead absorption from the gi tract. Iron deficiency, in addition, increases pica behavior. For levels > 45, DMSA (succimer) has the advantage of being oral. If > 70, two-drug therapy is recommended, and IV Ca-EDTA is added. If po succimer is not tolerated, a combination of im BAL and IV EDTA are given sequentially. Drug treatment of lead poisoning rare.
- Current management involves environmental inspection for the lead source; appropriate deleading if identified; move family to lead-free environment.
- EBLL that triggers a formal inspection varies from region to region depending on prevalence and resources.
- All families where children are identified should be given nutritional and housing hygiene guidance: picking up loose chips, vacuuming, and mopping areas where lead dust may accumulate all can reduce exposure.

15.6 Colic

General Ref

- *Pediatrics* 1998;102:e1282
- Ronald G. Barr, *Colic and Crying Syndromes in Infant*
- *Pediatr Rev* 2007;28:381–385

Def

- Paroxysmal crying (assumed to be intestinal in origin) in an infant between 2 wk and 4 months of age. Difficult to comfort.

- Parents typically describe abdominal distention, legs drawn up, flush face or pallor, sweating, cool hands and feet, difficult to comfort. Most commonly in late afternoon and evenings, with infant acting normally the rest of the d.

Pathophys

- Dominant theory: normal digestive processes lead to discomfort and a proportion of infants with more "intense" personalities cry "excessively" and are difficult to comfort; and therefore, more frequent smaller meals and frequent burping should help somewhat.
- Second theory: these infants miss constraint of womb environment, thus are aided by aggressive swaddling.
- Third theory: protein intolerance plays a role and switching to a hydrolysate is appropriate.
- Others subscribe to the reflux theory, and many infants with "colic" are tried on H2 blockers or PPIs.

Diff Dx

- Careful attention to H + P. If situation is more acute without hx of d to wk of recurrent crying (with normal behaviors between), consider possible path-ology. Conditions that cause paroxysmal infant crying can include hair tourniquets, incarcerated hernias, SVT, corneal abrasions, child abuse, and intussusception. Arching and spitting can suggest ge reflux. Consider protein sensitivities, infection.

Assessment

- No indicated tests unless H + P suggests some disease process.
- Most important variables to track are input (type of formula, stool and void pattern, spitting), weight gain, pattern of crying, ability to be soothed, unusual posturing, fever, respiratory symptoms, symmetric movement of extremities.

Rx

- Careful examination and reassurance with monitoring normal growth, attention to feeding practices, comfort measures.
- Breastfeeding mothers should avoid dairy products, chocolate, and "gassy" vegetables.
- In bottle-fed pts, formula changes are often done with variable results, although there are some limited data that support switching to a hydrolysate.
- Trials of H2 blockers or PPIs are often done for presumed "reflux" with little documentation.
- Probiotic use (*Lactobacillus reuteri*) is supported by one study, which showed impressive 90% improvement by 6 wk.
- Chiropractic and osteopathic manipulation have little supporting data. Herbal teas with fennel and/or chamomile are harmless and occasionally soothing, and there are some data that sucrose helps quiet the younger infants.
- Aggressive swaddling to constrain infant movements may work to imitate the intrauterine environment. Increasing physical contact with the parent ($\geq$ 3 hr of holding per d) augments its benefit.

15.7   Labial Adhesions (Synechia Vilvae)

General Ref

- *Arch Dis Child* 2007;92:268

General

- Labia minora adherent in the midline.
- May be partial or complete with just a pinhole orifice.
- Asymptomatic adhesions usually lyse spontaneously.
- If there is perineal irritation or diversion of urinary stream, treat with an estrogen cream (e.g., Premarin cream).

- Important to apply sparingly for short period to limit systemic absorption (breast bud formation side effect).
- Very rarely active separation under anesthesia is required (failed medical therapy due to thick adhesions).

15.8   Amblyopia and Strabismus (Squint)

General Ref

- *Pediatrics* 2003;111:902–907
- *Pediatrics* 2008;122:1401–1404

General

- Newborns' vision is limited at birth with a well-developed peripheral retina but immature fovea. Fovea is mature by 4 yr.
- During the critical period of visual maturation, well-focused images on both the retina are necessary for the proper development of visual acuity.
- Anything impairing clear images will affect normal development of the optic pathway and visual cortex and may be amblyogenic.

Cause

- Cataracts, retinoblastoma, congenital infections, hypoxic ischemic encephalopathy, retinopathy of prematurity, optic nerve hypoplasia

Epidem

- Severe visual impairment 1 in 1000 live births, developed countries 50% cases genetic; in developing countries acquired causes such as infection more common

S+S

- Cortical visual impairment from cerebral damage: eye examination, pupillary responses may be normal.

- Visual impairment may present in infancy with any of the following:
  - Photophobia, nystagmus, squint
  - No red reflex (cataract)
  - White reflex (cataract, retinoblastoma, retinopathy of prematurity)
  - Lack of eye contact with parents, visual inattention: unable to fix and follow
  - Not smiling responsively by 6 wk

Amblyopia

- Potentially permanent loss of visual acuity from disuse or misuse during the critical period of development.
- Caused by any interference with visual development (e.g., strabismus, hemangioma, ptosis, cataract, refractive errors). Hypermetropia is the most common refractive error in young children; early correction essential to prevent amblyopia. Myopia uncommon in young children; less likely to cause amblyopia unless severe).
- Delay in treatment reduces the likelihood of normal vision and after 7 yr improvement unlikely.

Strabismus (Squint)

- Anomaly of ocular alignment.
- Due to failure to develop binocular vision (e.g., cataracts, refractive errors, retinoblastoma).
- Often intermittent and parents usually correct if they report deviation.
- There may be a positive family hx.
- Presentation of squint:
  - Latent: only apparent at certain times (e.g., fatigue, illness, stress).
  - Manifest: present all the time.

- Alternating: uses either eye for fixation while the other is deviated; as each eye used in turn, vision develops equally.
- Monocular: only one eye used for fixation, the other constantly deviates, risk of amblyopia in the deviated eye.
- Convergent: turns in.
- Divergent: turns out.
- Nonparalytic: common and includes most of congenital and infantile convergent squints. May be due to refractive errors. May require surgery. More common with neurodevelopmental delay and may be convergent (most common), divergent, or rarely vertical.
- Paralytic: rare and due to weakness or paralysis of one or more extraocular muscles. Congenital paralytic squints due to developmental defects of the cranial nerves, muscle disease, or congenital infection. Acquired paralytic squint usually occur with a serious pathologic process (e.g., brain tumor, CNS infection, neurodegenerative disease).

Course

- Assessment:
  - Ocular movements assessed to exclude paralytic squint.
  - Corneal light reflex: Light reflection should appear in the same position in both eyes.
  - Cover test: when a squint is present and the fixing eye is covered, the squinting eye moves to take up fixation.

Rx

- Any infant with a squint after 2–3 months should be referred to an ophthalmologist.
- Rapid onset paralytic squint; work up for a space-occupying lesion.

Principles of Rx

- Develop optimal vision for both eyes:
  - Correct underlying defects (e.g., cataract).

- Correct refractive errors with glasses.
- Treat any amblyopia with occlusion therapy.
- Achieve best ocular alignment:
  - Surgery may be required.
  - The longer the delay in treatment, the less chance of normal vision being obtained.

Chapter 16

Genetics

16.1 Tuberous Sclerosis Complex

General Ref
- *Lancet* 2008;372:657–668

Cause
- One-third autosomal dominant and two-thirds sporadic.
- Of sporadic form, TSC 2 mutation is 5 times more common.
- Of the familial forms, 50% TSC 1 mutation and 50% TSC 2 mutation.

Epidem
- 1 in 6000–10,000

Pathophys
- Disease of cell size dysregulation, multisystem involvement with large hamartomas

Sx
- Seizures with infantile spasms in infancy, mental retardation, and autism

Si
- See major and minor features in Table 16.1.

Dx

- Definite: 2 major features or 1 major and 1 minor
- Probable: 1 major feature or 2 minor
- Possible: 1 major or 2 or more minor.

Course

- Variable

Complications

- Seizures 75–90%; the earlier the onset the more likely mental retardation will occur; ventricular obstruction and hydro-cephalus, cardiac involvement, renal failure (*N Engl J Med* 1998;338:1886), honeycombing of lung.

Lab

- EEG awake and sleep; CT/MRI head shows calcified tumors, gliomas.

Table 16.1 Tuberous Sclerosis Complex

Major Features	Minor Features
Shagreen patch	Dental pits
Cortical tubers	Gingival fibromas
Subependymal nodules	Bone cysts
Facial angiofibromas	Renal cysts
Ungual/periungual fibromas	Confetti skin lesions
Cardiac rhabdomyomas	Nonrenal hamartomas
Renal angiomyolipomas	Hamartomatous rectal polyps
Hypomelanotic macules > 3	Retinal achromatic patch
Retinal hamartomas	Cerebral white matter migration lines
Subependymal giant cell astrocytomas	
Pulmonary lymphangioleiomyomatosis	

Rx

- Seizures:
  - Medical treatment: antiepileptic drugs, in infantile spasms vigabatrin or adrenocorticotropic hormone (*Epilepsia* 1998;39(2):233–234; *Epilepsia* 2004;45(5):410–423).
  - Surgical treatment: cortical resection, corpus callosotomy.
  - Manage complications.

16.2   Neurofibromatosis Type 1

General Ref

- *Pediatrics* 2000;105:608–614
- *JAMA* 1997;2(278):51–57

Cause

- Autosomal dominant; 50% sporadic

Epidem

- Incidence: 1 in 3000–3500; prevalence: 1 in 100,000

Pathophys

- NF1 gene localized to chromosome 17q11.2 (*Am J Hum Genet* 1989;44:20–24)

S+S

- Variable depending on site of involvement
- National Institute of Health diagnostic criteria: 2 or more are necessary for diagnosis, as shown in Table 16.2.

Course

- Variable

GENETICS

Table 16.2   Neurofibromatosis Type I Diagnostic Criteria

$\geq$ 6 café au lait spots: > 5 mm diameter prepubertal and > 15 mm diameter postpubertal

$\geq$ 2 neurofibromas or 1 plexiform neurofibroma

Axillary or inguinal freckling

Optic glioma

$\geq$ 2 iris hamartomas (Lisch nodules)

Typical osseous lesion (e.g., sphenoid dysplasia, tibial dysplasia)

Affected first-degree relative

Complications

- Malignancy: chronic myeloblastic leukemia in children (*N Engl J Med* 1997;336:1713), learning disabilities, cerebrovascular disease, hypertension, pheochromocytomas, renal artery stenosis, scoliosis; 10% of plexiform neurofibromas undergo malignant change in 2nd to 3rd decade of life.

Lab/Imaging

- Diagnosis clinical. Test for complications and clinical symptoms as appropriate.
- DNA testing in atypical cases
- MRI not routine. UBOs(unidentified bright objects) seen especially in 8–16 yr age group

Rx

- Annual: clinical exam, blood pressure, ophthalmology evaluation, scoliosis screening (*Ann Neurol* 2007).
- Managed by a multidisciplinary team.
- Rx complications. Interventions are palliative and supportive.

16.3   Neurofibromatosis Type 2

Cause

- Autosomal dominant; 50% sporadic

Epidem:

- Improved clinical and molecular diagnostic techniques have resulted in syndrome being recognized more frequently. (*Otol Neurotol* 2005;26(1):93–97, *Am J Med Genet A* 2010; 152A(2):327–332)

Pathophys

- NF2 gene localized to chromosome 22q11.2

Sx

- Sensorineural hearing loss, vertigo, tinnitus, facial palsies, dysphagia, facial numbness (Daniel K. Onion, *Little Black Book of Family Medicine*)

Si

- See diagnostic criteria in Table 16.3.

Table 16.3   Diagnostic Criteria for Neurofibromatosis Type 2

Bilateral vestibular Schwannoma *or*

First-degree relative with neurofibromatosis type 2 + any 2 of the following:

- Meningioma
- Glioma
- Schwannoma
- Ependymoma
- Juvenile posterior subcapsular cataract

GENETICS

Course

- Onset: teens to 20s

Lab

- Brainstem auditory evoked responses 100% positive
  (*N Engl J Med* 1984;310:1740)

Xray

- MRI or CT with contrast

Rx

- Surgery (*N Engl J Med* 1998;339:1426)

16.4   Down Syndrome

General Ref

- *Pediatrics* 2001;107(2):442–449

Cause

- Genetic defect trisomy 21

Epidem

- Incidence (varies with age); overall 1 in 600–700 live births,
  M:F 1.3:1; most common autosomal chromosome abnormality causing mental retardation, spontaneous abortion in early
  pregnancy in 50% trisomy 21 fetuses

Pathophys

- 90–95% due to nondisjunction during egg or sperm formation
  resulting in a gamete with two 21st chromosomes, thus with
  conception genotype of complete trisomy 21.
- If nondisjunction occurs after fertilization, 2–4%, results in
  mosaicism: cell lines with and without extra chromosome 21.

- Complete or partial translocation of chromosome 21 genetic material to another chromosome occurs in 2–4%. In this case, if one of the parents carries a balanced translocation the risk of recurrence is much higher and genetic counseling should be offered.

S+S

- Feeding problems, snoring
- Brachycephaly, upslanting palpebral fissures, epicanthic folds, Brushfield spots on iris, single palmar crease, hypotonia, mental retardation, small nose with flat nasal bridge, high arched palate, delayed teeth eruption, wide gap between 1st and 2nd toes

Complications

- The following are more common in Down syndrome:
  - Congenital heart disease: ventricular septal defect, atrioventricular septal defect, patent ductus arteriosus, atrial septal defect, aberrant subclavian artery, tetralogy of Fallot
  - Gastrointestinal abnormalities: duodenal atresia, Hirschsprung disease, imperforate anus, Meckel diverticulum
  - Hematologic abnormalities: ALL, AML, transient myeloproliferative disorder
  - Thyroid disease: congenital hypothyroidism, hyperthyroidism
  - Cataracts, strabismus, nystagmus
  - Alzheimer disease: nearly all by age 40 yr
  - Mild to moderate MR (IQ 25–75)

Lab

- ECG within 1st month of life r/o cardiac malformation
- Auditory brainstem response within first 3 months of life to r/o out hearing loss.
- Routine maternal triple screen at 15–18 wk gestational age; if positive go on to amniocentesis and karyotyping.

- CBC in neonate to r/o transient myeloproliferative disorder and polycythemia
- Thyroid function tests
- Imaging: Echocardiogram within 1st month for congenital heart disease

Rx

- Prevention with screening. Treat specific complications.

16.5 Turner Syndrome

General Ref

- *J Clin Endocrinol Metab* 2007;92:10
- *Pediatrics* 1995;96:1166–1173

Cause

- Genetic mutation with 45XO (or XO/XX, rarely XO/XY) karyotype

Epidem

- 1 in 2000–2500 live born females; frequent finding in miscarriages

Pathophys

- Gonadal dysgenesis; most common sex chromosome aneuploidy

S+S

- Short stature (mean adult height: 142 cm), primary amenorrhea, normal intelligence.
- Lymphedema of hands and feet, widely spaced nipples. Shield-shaped chest, short 4th metacarpal, wide carrying angle, high arched palate, webbed neck, low posterior hairline, infertility,

hypothyroidism, excessive pigmented nevi, recurrent ear infections

Complications

- DM 2, Hashimoto thyroiditis, coarctation of the aorta, horse-shoe kidneys, duplicated ureters, renal aplasia, hypertension

Lab

- Low estrogen, increased LH and FSH

Xray

- Prenatal US may show associated renal anomalies.
- Renal US done at dx.
- Echocardiogram if congenital heart disease suspected.

Rx

- Routine BP screening.
- Thyroid function tests every 1–2 yr from the age of 10 yr.
- Routine developmental screening; use Turner syndrome growth charts.
- Short stature; refer to endocrinologist at 4 yr to consider growth hormone therapy. Final height can be increased with GH (*N Engl J Med* 1999;340:502–557).

16.6   Williams Syndrome

General Ref

- *Am J Hum Genet* 1995;57:49–53

Cause

- Genetic defect 7q11.23 deletion, including elastin gene ELN

GENETICS

Epidem

- Incidence: 1 in 20,000

Pathophys

- Incompletely understood

S+S

- Mild mental retardation, hypercalcemia, serrated teeth, carp-shaped mouth, elfin facies, hypertelorism, short stature, microcephaly, long neck, small nails, prematurely aging skin, cocktail party chatter, hypersensitivity to sound

Complications

- Supravalvular AS, peripheral pulmonary artery stenosis, renal artery stenosis with renovascular hypertension, hypercalcemia-induced nephrocalcinosis.

Xray

- Echocardiogram, renal US at diagnosis

Lab

- Serum calcium at dx; then every 2 yr
- Urine calcium-to-creatinine ratio every 2 yr
- Renal function and urinalysis every 2 yr

Rx

- Treat complications: cardiology and nephrology consults as appropriate
- Use William syndrome growth charts. Consider endocrinology referral to discuss growth hormone therapy if short stature
- Dental evaluation and orthodontist referral at 8 yr of age
- Early referral for audiologic evaluation, speech therapy, occupational therapy, and physical therapy

- Neuropsychological screening as part of developmental screening

16.7 Klinefelter Syndrome

General Ref

- *J Clin Endocrinol Metab* 2003;88:622–626

Cause

- Sex chromosome aneuploidy karyotype 47XXY, sporadic inheritance

Epidem

- 1 in 600 newborn males

Pathophys

- 47XXY karyotype from nondisjunction of the sex chromosomes, associated with advanced parental age

S+S

- Sexual immaturity, infertility
- Tall and slim, gynecomastia with increased risk of male breast cancer, cryptorchidism, azoospermia and infertility, normal to low IQ (generally 10 points below siblings), mild developmental and behavioral problems

Complications

- Breast cancer (*N Engl J Med* 1980;303:795), ADHD more common

Lab

- LH and FSH, testosterone

Rx

- Consider testosterone therapy.
- Paternity through sperm aspiration and in vitro fertilization (*N Engl J Med* 1998;338:588).
- Regular breast exam in adulthood, consider mastectomy for gynecomastia.
- Monitor for learning disabilities and early intervention.

16.8 Marfan Syndrome

General Ref

- *Lancet* 2005;366:1965–1976

Cause

- Autosomal dominant; 15% sporadic

Pathophys

- Mutation in the fibrillin 1 (*FBN1*) gene on chromosome 15

S+S

- Frequent joint dislocations from minor injuries, myopia, tall, plus family hx
- Arm span > height (dolichostenomelia), arachnodactyly, lens dislocation upward, high arched palate, joint laxity, scoliosis, pes planus, striae of skin

Course

- Death in early 30s due to aortic dissection, aortic or mitral insufficiency

Complications

- Aortic root dilation and dissection, mitral valve prolapse, pneumothorax

Xray

- Chest Xray, echocardiogram

Rx

- Beta-blocker to keep exercise heart rate < 100 bpm slows disease progression (*N Engl J Med* 1994;330:1335).
- In a small cohort study, the use of angiotensin receptor blocker therapy in pts with Marfan syndrome significantly slowed the rate of progressive aortic-root dilation (*N Engl J Med* 2008;358: 2787–2795).

16.9   Fetal Alcohol Syndrome

General Ref

- *Obstet Gynecol* 2005;106:1059–1064

Cause

- Alcohol use during pregnancy. Safe level has not been established; complete abstinence recommended.

Epidem

- 1–3 infants per 1000 live births

Pathophys

- Alcohol teratogenesis, alteration in neuronal numbers, heterotopias, decreases in white matter, problems with dendritic proliferation

S+S

- Irritability, hyperactivity, average IQ
- Microcephaly, short palpebral fissure, short nose, smooth philtrum, thin upper lip, maxillary hypoplasia, small distal phalanges, small 5th fingernail, VSD, auricular septal defect

GENETICS

- Less common: microphthalmia, cleft lip/palate, webbed neck, short neck, cardiac malformations, renal malformations

Complications

- High risk for neglect, abuse

Rx

- Early recognition and close follow-up

16.10   Velocardiofacial Syndrome

General Ref

- *J Pediatr* 2001;139:715–723
- *Am J Med Genet A* 2006;140:906

Cause

- Autosomal dominant

Epidem

- 1 in 4000 live births

Pathophys

- Deletion in chromosome 22q11

S+S

- Velo: cleft palate: submucous or overt; hypernasal speech due to weak pharyngeal muscles
- Cardio: VSD, tetralogy of Fallot, transposition of the great vessels, conotruncal heart disease, right-sided aortic arch
- Facial: long vertical face, micrognathia, prominent nose, small abnormal ears, narrow eyes
- Other: hypotonia, feeding problems, transient neonatal hypocalcemia, T-cell dysfunction, learning disabilities, developmental delay, renal abnormalities

Lab

- Fluorescent in-situ hybridization (FISH)
- CBC with lymphocyte subsets
- Total immunoglobulins
- Serum calcium

Imaging

- Echocardiogram
- Renal US

Rx

- ENT referral for palatial and pharyngeal problems
- Cardiology referral
- Speech therapy
- Neuropsychiatric evaluation

16.11   Friedreich Ataxia

General Ref

- *Arch Neurol* 2008;65(10):1296–1303

Cause

- Autosomal recessive.
- Most common hereditary ataxia.
- Caused by expansion of GAA trinucleotide repeat located on frataxin gene on chromosome 9q13.
- Larger GAA expansions, particularly on the smaller allele, correlate with earlier age at onset, shorter times to loss of ambulation, a greater frequency of cardiomyopathy, and loss of reflexes in the upper limbs (*N Engl J Med* 1996;335(16):1169–1175).

GENETICS

Pathophys

- Frataxin protein is a mitochondrial protein that plays a role in iron homeostasis.
- Overexpression of frataxin increases cellular antioxidant defense through activation of glutathione peroxidase and elevation of reduced thiols.
- Pts with Friedreich ataxia have impairment of enzymatic antioxidants.

S+S

- Onset < 25 yr of age. Progressive ataxia, absent lower extremity reflexes, axonal and sensory neuropathy, dysarthria and areflexia

Lab

- Motor nerve conduction studies usually normal.
- MRI may show spinal cord and cerebellar atrophy.
- Genetic testing confirms dx.

16.12   Spina Bifida

General Ref

- *N Engl J Med* 1999;341:1509

Cause

- Neural tube defect due to failure of normal fusion of neural plate to form the neural tube. Defects of increasing severity:
  - Spina bifida occulta, which has no clinical significance
  - Meningocele, meningomyelocele, and myelocele
- Most cases idiopathic; maternal hypervitaminosis A > 10,000 IU daily especially 1st trimester (*N Engl J Med* 1995;333:1369)

Epidemiol

- 1 in 1000 births in United States; risk doubled with maternal obesity (JAMA 1996;275:1089, 1093)

S+S

- Minor defects: overlying skin defect such as hair tuft, lipoma or small dermal sinus usually in the lumbar region
- Obvious open defect: skin defect, exposed neural plate, or cord protected by pia arachnoid.
- Associated CNS abnormalities such as hydrocephalus

Course

- Meningocele good prognosis with surgical repair
- Myelomeningocele associated with many problems. Poor prognosis if severe hydrocephalus, severe kyphosis, poor social support.

Complications

- Hydrocephalus
- Orthopedic problems: kyphoscoliosis, talipes
- Bladder/bowel problems: neuropathic bladder, rectal prolapse
- Variable: leg paralysis, sensory loss

Lab

- Prenatal screening at 15–18 wk gestational age: alpha feto-protein (AFP), human chorionic gonadotropin, and estriol levels.
- Elevated maternal AFP associated with increased maternal loss

Rx

- Folic acid > 4 mg daily dramatically decreases neural tube defects (JAMA 1995;274:1698; N Engl J Med 1998;338:1060)

GENETICS

- Immediate management:
  - Prone position
  - Cover and prevent fecal soiling of exposed neural tissue
  - Broad-spectrum antibiotics
  - Intermittent urinary catheterization
- Surgery:
  - Formal closure of defect
  - Ventricular shunt for hydrocephalus
  - Orthopedic procedures may be required

Chapter 17

Childhood Immunizations

General Ref

- Centers for Disease Control and Prevention (CDC). Recommended immunization schedules for persons ages 0–18 years—United States, 2009.
- *MMWR* 2009;57(51 and 52):38 with modifications from CDC.
- Updated recommendations of the Advisory Committee on Immunization Practices (ACIP) regarding routine poliovirus vaccination.
- *MMWR* 2009;58:829.
- Daniel K. Onion, *Little Black Book of Family Practice*

General Rules

- Give when due, as long as temperature ≤ 100°F (37.7°C) (*JAMA* 1996;275:704; *JAMA* 1991;265:2095).
- Slight increase in febrile seizures with measles, mumps, rubella (MMR) without long-term sequelae (*JAMA* 2004;292:351).
- Give diphtheria-tetanus, diphtheria, pertussis, tetanus, Hib and Hepatitis B im; give MMR sc.
- Hib is for MSD 3-shot series; other types require additional dose at 6 months, but using any of the 3 available Hib vaccines at 2, 4, 6, and 12–15 months is OK (*JAMA* 1995;273:849).
- Conjugate pneumococcal 7-valent vaccine in children; almost 30% decrease in rates of invasive pneumococcal

disease in infants 0–90 d old since introduction
(JAMA 2006;295:1668).

- Hepatitis A killed vaccine series (2 shots, 6+ months apart)
  sometime between age 1 and adult.
- Meningococcal C vaccine for infants at 2, 3, and 4 months
  works but decreases immunogenicity of other vaccines
  (JAMA 2005;293:1751).
- Egg allergies not a contraindication to measles vaccination
  (*N Engl J Med* 1995;332:1262).
- Few to none now contain mercury preservative.

Table 17.1

Recommended Immunization Schedule for Persons Aged 0 Through 6 Years—United States • 2010

For those who fall behind or start late, see the catch-up schedule

Vaccine ▼ Age ▶	Birth	1 month	2 months	4 months	6 months	12 months	15 months	18 months	19-23 months	2-3 years	4-6 years
Hepatitis B [1]	HepB	HepB			HepB						
Rotavirus [2]			RV	RV	RV						
Diphtheria, Tetanus, Pertussis [3]			DTaP	DTaP	DTaP		DTaP				DTaP
Haemophilus influenzae type b [4]			Hib	Hib	Hib4	Hib					
Pneumococcal [5]			PCV	PCV	PCV	PCV				PPSV	
Inactivated Poliovirus [6]			IPV	IPV	IPV						IPV
Influenza [7]					Influenza (Yearly)						
Measles, Mumps, Rubella [8]						MMR			see footnote 8		MMR
Varicella [9]						Varicella			see footnote 9		Varicella
Hepatitis A [10]						HepA (2 doses)				HepA Series	
Meningococcal [11]										MCV	

Range of recommended ages for all children except certain high-risk groups

Range of recommended ages for certain high-risk groups

This schedule includes recommendations in effect as of December 15, 2009. Any dose not administered at the recommended age should be administered at a subsequent visit, when indicated and feasible. The use of a combination vaccine generally is preferred over separate injections of its equivalent component vaccines. Considerations should include provider assessment, patient preference, and the potential for adverse events. Providers should consult the relevant Advisory Committee on Immunization Practices statement for detailed recommendations: http://www.cdc.gov/vaccines/pubs/acip-list.htm reported to the Vaccine Adverse Event Reporting System (VAERS) at http://www.vaers.hhs.gov or by telephone, 800-822-7967.

(continued)

Table 17.1 (continued)

1. Hepatitis B vaccine (HepB). (Minimum age: birth)

At birth:

- Administer monovalent HepB to all newborns before hospital discharge.
- If mother is hepatitis B surface antigen (HBsAg)-positive, administer HepB and 0.5 mL of hepatitis B immune globulin (HBIG) within 12 hours of birth.
- If mother's HBsAg status is unknown, administer HepB within 12 hours of birth. Determine mother's HBsAg status as soon as possible and, if HBsAg-positive, administer HBIG (no later than age 1 week).

After the birth dose:

- The HepB series should be completed with either monovalent HepB or a combination vaccine containing HepB. The second dose should be administered at age 1 or 2 months. Monovalent HepB vaccine should be used for doses administered before age 24 weeks. The final dose should be administered no earlier than age 24 weeks.
- Infants born to HBsAg-positive mothers should be tested for HBsAg and antibody to HBsAg 1 to 2 months after completion of at least 3 doses of the HepB series, at age 9 through 18 months (generally at the next well-child visit).
- Administration of 4 doses of HepB to infants is permissible when a combination vaccine containing HepB is administered after the birth dose. The fourth dose should be administered no earlier than age 24 weeks.

2. Rotavirus vaccine (RV). (Minimum age: 6 weeks)

- Administer the first dos at age 6 through 14 weeks (maximum age: 14 weeks 6 days). Vaccination should not be initiated for infants aged 15 weeks 0 days or older.
- The maximum age for the final dose in the series is 6 months 0 days.
- If Rotarix is administered at ages 2 and 4 months, a dose at 6 months is not indicated.

3. Diphtheria and tetanus toxoids and acellular pertussis vaccine (DTaP). (Minimum age: 6 weeks)

- The fourth dose may be administered as early as age 12 months, provided at least 6 months have elapsed since the third dose.
- Administer the final dose in the series at age 4 through 6 years.

4. *Haemophilus influenzae* type b conjugate vaccine (Hib). (Minimum age: 6 weeks)

- If PRP-OMP (PedvaxHIB or Comvax [HepB-Hib]) is administered at ages 2 and 4 months, a dose at age 6 months is not indicated.
- TriHiBit (DTaP/Hib) and Hiberix (PRP-T) should not be used for doses at ages children aged 12 months through 4 years. See *MMWR* 1997;46(No. RR-8).

5. Pneumococcal vaccine. (Minimum age: 6 weeks for pneumococcal conjugate vaccine [PCV]; 2 years for pneumococcal polysaccharide vaccine [PPSV])

- PCV is recommended for all children aged younger than 5 years. Administer 1 dose of PCV to all healthy children aged 24 through 59 months who are not completely vaccinated for their age.
- Administer PPSV 2 or more months after last dose of PCV to children aged 2 years or older with certain underlying medical conditions, including a cochlear implant.

6. Inactivated poliovirus vaccine (IPV). (Minimum age: 6 weeks)

- The final dose in the series should be administered on or after the fourth birthday and at least 6 months following the previous dose.
- If 4 doses are administered prior to age 4 years a fifth dose should be administered at age 4 through 6 years. See *MMWR* 2009;58(30):829-30.

7. Influenza vaccine (seasonal). (Minimum age: 6 months for trivalent inactivated influenza vaccine [TIV]; 2 years for live, attenuated influenza vaccine [LAIV])

- Administer annually to children aged 2 through 6 years (i.e., those who do not have underlying medical conditions that predispose them to influenza complications), either LAIV or TIV may be used, except LAIV should not be given to children aged 2 though 4 years who have had wheezing in the past 12 months.

- Children receiving TIV should receive 0.25 mL if aged 6 through 35 months or 0.5 mL if aged 3 years or older.
- Administer 2 doses (separated by at least 4 weeks) to children aged younger than 9 years who are receiving influenza vaccine for the first time or who were vaccinated for the first time during the previous influenza season but only received one dose.
- For recommendations for use of influenza A (H1N1) 2009 monavalent vaccine see *MMWR* 2009;58(No.RR-10).

8. Measles, mumps and rubella vaccine (MMR). (Minimum age: 12 months)

- Administer the second dose routinely at age 4 through 6 years. However, the second dose may be administered before age 4, provided at least 28 days have elapsed since the first dose.

9. Varicella vaccine. (Minimum age: 12 months)

- Administer the second dose routinely at age 4 through 6 years. However, the second dose may be administered before age 4, provided at least 3 months have elasped since the first dose.
- For children aged 12 months through 12 years the minimum interval between doses is 3 months. However, if the second dose

was administered at least 28 days after the first dose, it can be accepted as valid.

10. Hepatitis A vaccine (HepA). (Minimum age: 12 months)

- Administer to all children aged 1 year (i.e., aged 12 through 23 months). Administer 2 doses at least 6 months apart.
- Children not fully caccinated by age 2 years can be caccinated at subsequent visits.
- HepA also is recommended for older children who live in areas where vaccination programs target older children, who are at increased risk for infection, or for whom immunity against hepatitis A is desired.

11. Meningococcal vaccine. (Minimum age: 2 years for meningo coccal conjugate vaccine [MCV4] and for meningococcal polysaccharide vaccine [MPCV4])

- Administer MCV4 to children aged 2 through 10 years with persistent complement component deficiency, anatomic or functional asplenia, and certain other conditions placing them at high risk.
- Administer MCV4 to children previously vaccinated with MCV4 or MPSV4 after 3 years if first dose administered at age 2 through 6 years. See *MMWR* 2009;58:1042–3.

The Recommended Immunization Schedules for Persons Aged 0 through 18 Years are approved by the Advisory Committee on Immunization Practices (http://www.cdc.gov/vaccines/recs/acip), the American Academy of Pediatrics (http://www.aap.org), and the American Academy of Family Physicians (http://www.aafp.org). Department of Health and Human Services • Centers for Disease Control and Prevention

Table 17.2

Recommended Immunization Schedule for Persons Aged 7 Through 18 Years—United States • 2010

For those who fall behind or start late, see the schedule below and the catch-up schedule

Vaccine ▼ / Age ►	7–10 years	11–12 years	13–18 years
Tetanus, Diphtheria, Pertussis [1]		Tdap	Tdap
Human Papillomavirus [2]	see footnote 2	HPV (3 doses)	HPV series
Meningococcal [3]	MCV	MCV	MCV
Influenza [4]	Influenza (Yearly)		
Pneumococcal [5]		PPSV	
Hepatitis A [6]		HepA Series	
Hepatitis B [7]		Hep B Series	
Inactivated Poliovirus [8]		IPV Series	
Measles, Mumps, Rubella [9]		MMR Series	
Varicella [10]		Varicella Series	

Range of recommended ages for all children except certain high-risk groups

Range of recommended ages for catch-upimmunization

Range of recommended ages for certain high-risk groups

This schedule includes recommendations in effect as of December 15, 2009. Any dose not administered at the recommended age should be administered at a subsequent visit, when indicated and feasible. The use of a combination vaccine generally is preferred over separate injections of its equivalent component vaccines. Considerations should include provider assessment, patient preference, and the potential for adverse events. Providers should consult the relevant Advisory Committee on Immunization Practices statement for detailed recommendations: http://www.cdc.gov/vaccines/pubs/ acip-list.htm. Clinically significant adverse events that follow immunization should be reported to the Vaccine Adverse Event Reporting System (VAERS) at http://www.vaers.hhs.gov or by telephone, 800-822-7967.

1. **Tetanus and diphtheria toxoids and acellular pertussis vaccine** (Tdap). (Minimum age: 10 years for Boostrix and 11 years for Adacel)

- Administer at age 11 or 12 years for those who have completed the recommended childhood DTP/DTaP vaccination series and have not received a tetanus and diphtheria toxoid (Td) booster dose.
- Persons aged 13 through 18 years who have not received Tdap should receive a dose.
- A 5-year interval from the last Td dose is encouraged when Tdap is used as a booster dose; however, a shorter interval may be used if pertussis immunity is needed.

2. **Human papillomavirus vaccine (HPV).** (Minimum age: 9 years)

- Two HPV vaccines are licensed: a quadrivalent vaccine (HPV4) for the prevention of cervical, vaginal and vulvar cancers (in females) and genital warts (in females and males), and a bivalent vaccine (HPV2) for the prevention of cervical cancers in females.
- HPV vaccines are most effective for both males and females when given before exposure to HPV through sexual contact.
- HPV4 or HPV2 is recommended for the prevention of cervical precancers and cancers in females.
- HPV4 is recommended for the prevention of cervical, vaginal and vulvar precancers and cancers and genital warts in females.
- Administer the first dose to females at age 11 or 12 years.
- Administer the second dose 1 to 2 months after the first dose and the third dose 6 months after the first dose (at least 24 weeks after the first dose).
- Administer the series to females at age 13 through 18 years if not previously vaccinated.
- HPV4 may be administered in a 3-dose series to males aged 9 through 18 years to reduce their likelihood of acquiring genital warts.

3. **Meningococcal conjugate vaccine (MCV4).**

- Administer at age 11 or 12 years, or at age 13 through 18 years if not previously vaccinated.

- Administer to previously unvaccinated college freshmen living in a dormitory.
- Administer MCV4 to children aged 2 through 10 years with persistent complement component deficiency, anatomic or functional asplenia, or certain other conditions placing them at high risk.
- Administer to children previously vaccinated with MCV4 or MPSV4 who remain at increased risk after 3 years (if first dose administered at age 2 through 6 years) or after 5 years (if first dose administered at age 7 years or older). Persons whose only risk factor is living in on-campus housing are not recommended to receive an additional dose. See MMWR 2009;58:1042-3.

4. **Influenza vaccine (seasonal).**

- Administer annually to children aged 6 months through 18 years.
- For healthy nonpregnant persons aged 7 through 18 years (i.e., those who do not have underlying medical conditions that predispose them to influenza complications), either LAIV or TIV may be used.
- Administer 2 doses (separated by at least 4 weeks) to children aged younger than 9 years who are receiving influenza vaccine for the first time or who were vaccinated for the first time during the previous influenza season but only received 1 dose.
- For recommendations for use of influenza A (H1N1) 2009 monovalent vaccine. See MMWR 2009;58(No. RR-10)

5. **Pneumococcal polysaccharide vaccine (PPSV).**

- Administer to children with certain underlying medical conditions, including a cochlear implant. A single revaccination should be administered after 5 years to children with functional or anatomic asplenia or an immunocompromising condition. See MMWR 1997;46(No. RR-8).

6. **Hepatitis A vaccine (HepA).**

- Administer 2 doses at least 6 months apart.
- HepA is recommended for children older than 23 months of age who live in areas where vaccination programs target older children or who are at increased risk for infection or for whom immunity against hepatitis A is desired.

(continued)

Table 17.2 *(continued)*

7. Hepatitis B vaccine (HepB).

- Administer the 3-dose series to those not previously vaccinated.
- A 2-dose series (separated by at least 4 months) of adult formulation Recombivax HB is licensed for children aged 11 through 15 years.

8. Inactivated poliovirus vaccine (IPV).

- The final dose in the series should be administered on or after the fourth birthday and at least 6 months following the previous dose.
- If both OPV and IPV were administered as part of a series, a total of 4 doses should be administered, regardless of the child's current age.

9. Measles, mumps, and rubella vaccine (MMR).

- If not previously vaccinated, administer 2 doses or the second dose for those who have received only 1 dose, with at least 28 days between doses.

10. Varicella vaccine.

- For persons aged 7 through 18 years without evidence of immunity (see *MMWR* 2007;56[No. RR-4]), administer 2 doses if not previously vaccinated or the second dose if only 1 dose has been administered.
- For persons aged 7 through 12 years, the minimum interval between doses is 3 months. However, if the second dose was administered at least 28 days after the first dose, it can be accepted as valid.
- For persons aged 13 years and older, the minimum interval between doses is 28 days.

The Recommended Immunization Schedules for Persons Aged 0 through 18 Years are approved by the
Advisory Committee on Immunization Practices (http://www.cdc.gov/vaccines/recs/acip),
the American Academy of Pediatrics (http://www.aap.org),
and the American Academy of Family Physicians (http://www.aafp.org).
Department of Health and Human Services • Centers for Disease Control and Prevention

Table 17.3

Catch-up Immunization Schedule for Persons Aged 4 Months Through 18 Years Who Start Late or Who Are More Than 1 Month Behind—United States • 2010

The table below provides catch-up schedules and minimum intervals between doses for children whose vaccinations have been delayed. A vaccine series does not need to be restarted, regardless of the time that has elapsed between doses. Use the section appropriate for the child's age.

		PERSONS AGED 4 MONTHS THROUGH 6 YEARS			
		Minimum Interval Between Doses			
Vaccine	Minimum Age for Dose 1	Dose 1 to Dose 2	Dose 2 to Dose 3	Dose 3 to Dose 4	Dose 4 to Dose 5
Hepatitis B[1]	Birth	4 weeks	8 weeks (and at least 16 weeks after first dose)		
Rotavirus[3]	6 weeks	4 weeks	4 weeks[2]		
Diphtheria, Tetanus, Pertussis[3]	6 weeks	4 weeks	4 weeks	6 months	6 months[3]
Haemophilus influenzae type b[4]	6 weeks	4 weeks if first dose administered at younger than age 12 months 8 weeks (as final dose) if first dose administered at age 12-14 months No further doses needed if first dose administered at age 15 months or older	4 weeks[4] if current age is younger than 12 months 8 weeks (as final dose)[4] If current age is 12 months or older and first dose administered at younger than age 12 months and second dose administered at younger than 15 months No further doses needed if previous dose administered at age 15 months or older	8 weeks (as final dose) This dose only necessary for children aged 12 months through 59 months who received 3 doses before age 12 months	

(continued)

Table 17.3 (continued)

Pneumococcal[5]	6 weeks	**4 weeks** if first dose administered at younger than age 12 months **8 weeks (as final dose for healthy children)** if first dose administered at age 12 months or older or current age 24 through 59 months **No further doses needed** for healthy children if first dose administered at age 24 months or older	**4 weeks** if current age is younger than 12 months **8 weeks (as final dose for healthy children)** if current age is 12 months or older **No further doses needed** for healthy children if previous dose administered at age 24 months or older	**8 weeks (as final dose)** This dose only necessary for children aged 12 months through 59 months who received 3 doses before age 12 months or for high risk children who received 3 doses at any age
Inactive Poliovirus[6]	6 weeks	**4 weeks**	**4 weeks**	**6 months**
Measles, Mumps, Rubella[7]	12 months	**4 weeks**		
Varicella[8]	12 months	**3 months**		
Hepatitis A[9]	12 months	**6 months**		
PERSONS AGED 7 THROUGH 18 YEARS				
Tetanus, Diphtheria/ Tetanus, Diphtheria, Pertussis[10]	7 years[10]	**4 weeks**	**4 weeks** if first dose administered at younger than age 12 months **6 months** if first dose administered at 12 months or older	**6 months** if first dose administered at younger than age 12 months
Human Papillomavirus[11]	9 years	Routine dosing intervals are recommended[11]		
Hepatitis A[9]	12 months	**6 months**		

Hepatitis B[1]	Birth	4 weeks	8 weeks (and at least 16 weeks after first dose)	6 months
Inactivated Poliovirus[6]	6 weeks	4 weeks	4 weeks	6 months
Measles, Mumps, Rubella[7]	12 months	4 weeks	4 weeks	
Varicella[8]	12 months	3 months if person is younger than age 13 years / 4 weeks if person is aged 13 years or older		

1. Hepatitis B vaccine (HepB).

- Administer the 3-dose series to those not previously vaccinated.
- A 2-dose series (separated by at least 4 months) of adult formulation Recombivax HB is licensed for children aged 11 through 15 years.

2. Rotavirus vaccine (RV).

- The maximum age for the first dose is 14 weeks 6 days. Vaccination should not be initiated for infants aged 15 weeks 0 days or older.
- The maximum age for the final dose in the series is 8 months 0 days.
- If Rotarix was administered for the first and second doses, a third dose is not indicated.

3. Diphtheria and tetanus toxoids and acellular pertussis vaccine (DTaP).

- The fifth dose is not necessary if the fourth dose was administered at age 4 years or older.

4. Haemophilus influenzae type b conjugate vaccine (Hib).

- Hib vaccine is not generally recommended for persons aged 5 years or older. No efficacy data are available on which to base a recommendation concerning use of Hib vaccine for older children and adults. However, studies suggest good immunogenicity in persons who have sickle cell disease, leukemia, or HIV infection, or who have had a splenectomy; administering 1 dose of Hib vaccine to these persons who have not previously received Hib vaccine is not contraindicated.
- If the first 2 doses were PRP-OMP (PedvaxHIB or Comvax), and administered at age 11 months or younger, the third (and final) dose should be administered at age 12 through 15 months and at least 8 weeks after the second dose.
- If the first dose was administered at age 7 through 11 months, administer the second dose at least 4 weeks later and a final dose at age 12 through 15 months.

(continued)

Childhood Immunizations **353**

Table 17.3 *(continued)*

5. Pneumococcal vaccine.
- Administer 1 dose of pneumococcal conjugate vaccine (PCV) to all healthy children aged 24 through 59 months who have not received at least 1 dose of PCV on or after age 12 months.
- For children aged 24 through 59 months with underlying medical conditions, administer 1 dose of PCV if 3 doses were received previously or administer 2 doses of PCV at least 8 weeks apart if fewer than 3 doses were received previously.
- Administer pneumococcal polysaccharide vaccine (PPSV) to children aged 2 years or older with certain underlying medical conditions, including a cochlear implant, at least 8 weeks after the last dose of PCV.

6. Inactivated poliovirus vaccine (IPV).
- The final dose in the series should be administered on or after the fourth birthday and at least 6 months following the previous dose.
- A fourth dose is not necessary if the third dose was administered at age 4 years or older and at least 6 months following the previous dose.
- In the first 6 months of life, minimum age and minimum intervals are only recommended if the person is at risk for imminent exposure to circulating poliovirus travel to a polio-endemic region or during an outbreak).

7. Measles, mumps, and rubella vaccine (MMR).
- Administer the second dose routinely at age 4 through 6 years. However, the second dose may be administered before age 4, provided at least 28 days have elapsed since the first dose.
- If not previously vaccinated, administer 2 doses with at least 28 days between doses.

8. Varicella vaccine.
- Administer the second dose routinely at age 4 through 6 years. However, the second dose may be administered before age 4, provided at least 3 months have elapsed since the first dose.
- For persons aged 12 months through 12 years, the minimum interval between doses is 3 months. However, if the second dose was administered at least 28 days after the first dose, it can be accepted as valid.
- For persons aged 13 years and older, the minimum interval between doses is 28 days.

9. Hepatitis A vaccine (HepA).
- HepA is recommended for children older than 23 months who live in areas where vaccination programs target older children, who are at increased risk for infection, or for whom immunity against hepatitis A is desired.

10. Tetanus and diphtheria toxoids vaccine (Td) and tetanus and diphtheria toxoids and acellular pertussis vaccine (Tdap).
- Doses of DTaP are counted as part of the Td/Tdap series
- Tdap should be substituted for a single dose of Td in the catch-up series or as a booster for children aged 10 through 18 years; use Td for other doses.

11. Human papillomavirus vaccine (HPV).
- Administer the series to females at age 13 through 18 years if not previously vaccinated.
- Use recommended routine dosing intervals for series catch-up (i.e., the second and third doses should be administered at 1 to 2 and 6 months after the first dose). The minimum interval between the first and second doses is 4 weeks. The minimum interval between the second and third doses is 12 weeks, and the third dose should be administered at least 24 weeks after the first dose.

Information about reporting reactions after immunization is available online at http://www.vaers.hhs.gov or by telephone, 800-822-7967. Suspected cases of vaccine-preventable diseases should be reported to the state or local health department. Additional information, including precautions and contraindications for immunization, is available from the National Center for Immunization and Respiratory Diseases at http://www.cdc.gov/vaccines or telephone, 800-CDC-INFO (800-232-4636). Department of Health and Human Services • Centers for Disease Control and Prevention

Chapter 18

Growth Charts

Table 18.1   Length-for-Age Percentiles, Boys, Birth to 36 Months, CDC Growth Charts: United States

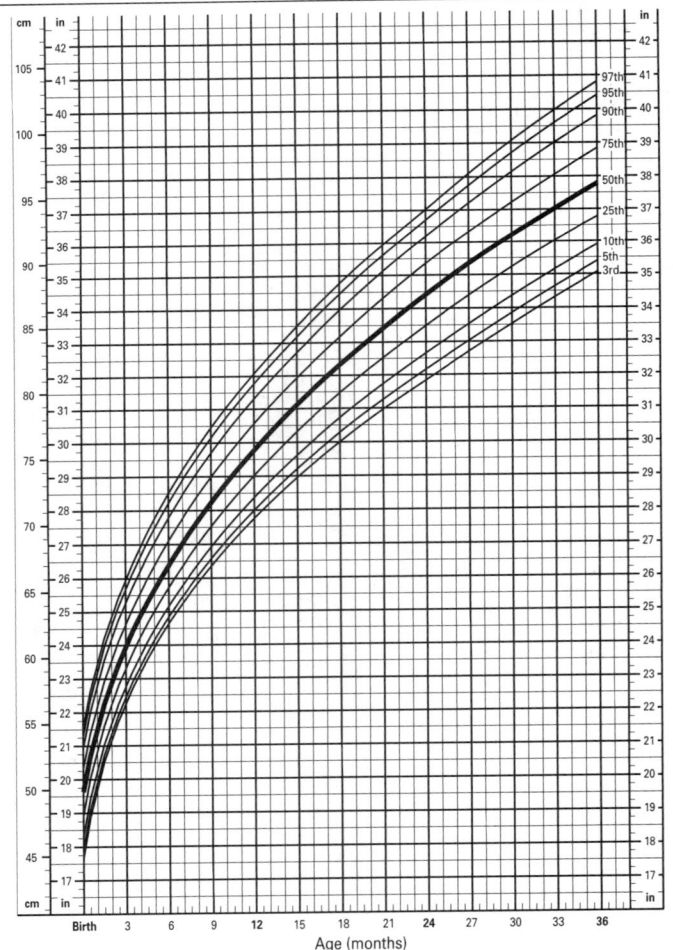

Source: Developed by the National Health Center for Health Statistics in collaboration with the National Center for Chronic Disease Prevention and Health Promotion (2000).

Table 18.2 Stature-for-Age Percentiles, Boys, 2 to 20 Years, CDC Growth Charts: United States

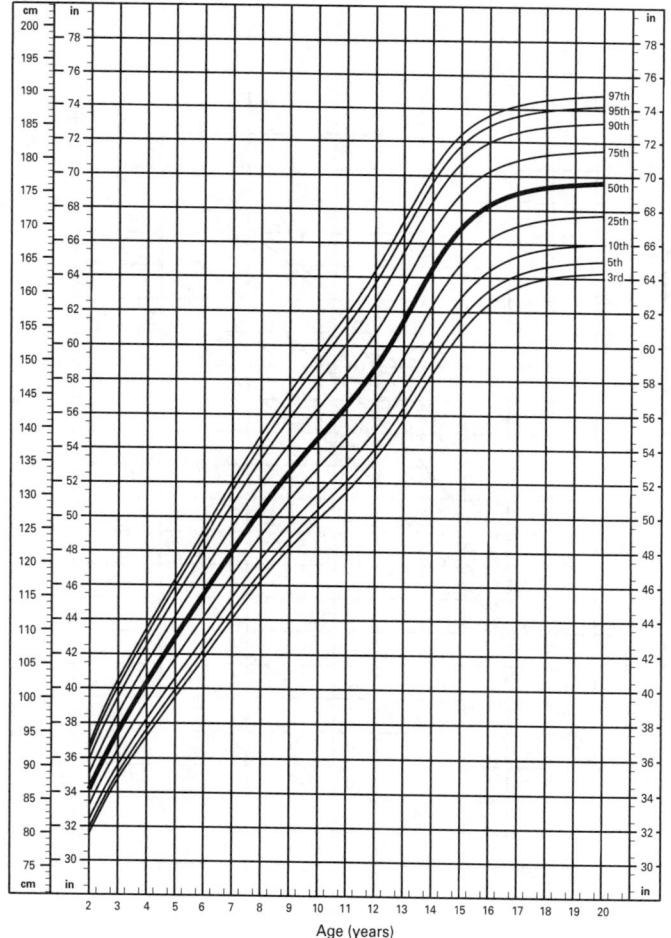

Source: Developed by the National Health Center for Health Statistics in collaboration with the National Center for Chronic Disease Prevention and Health Promotion (2000).

Table 18.3   Length-for-Age Percentiles, Girls, Birth to 36 Months, CDC Growth Charts: United States

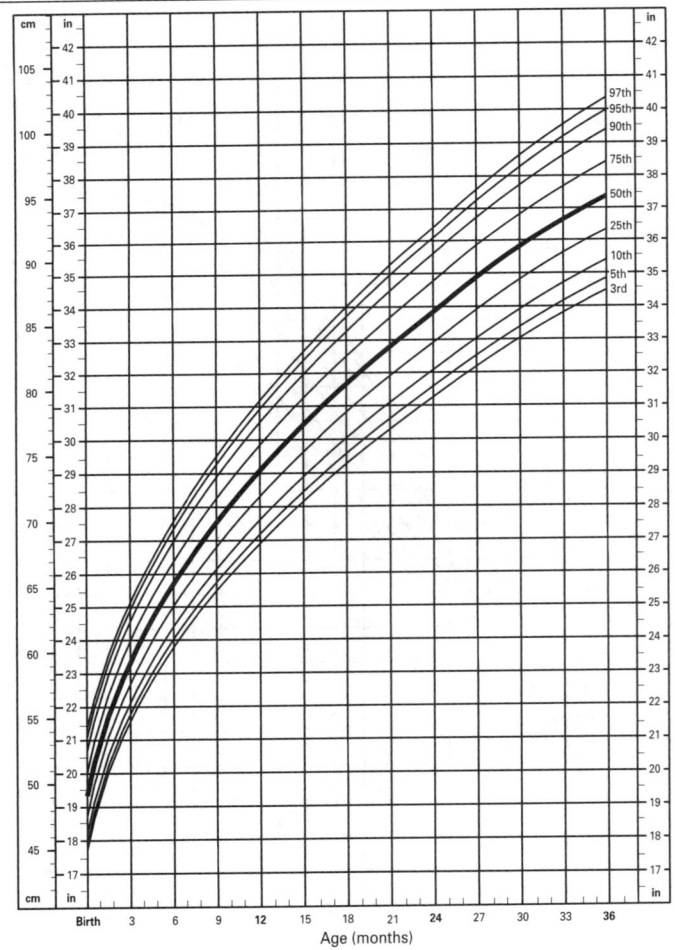

Source: Developed by the National Health Center for Health Statistics in collaboration with the National Center for Chronic Disease Prevention and Health Promotion (2000).

Table 18.4 Stature-for-Age Percentiles, Girls, 2 to 20 Years, CDC Growth Charts: United States

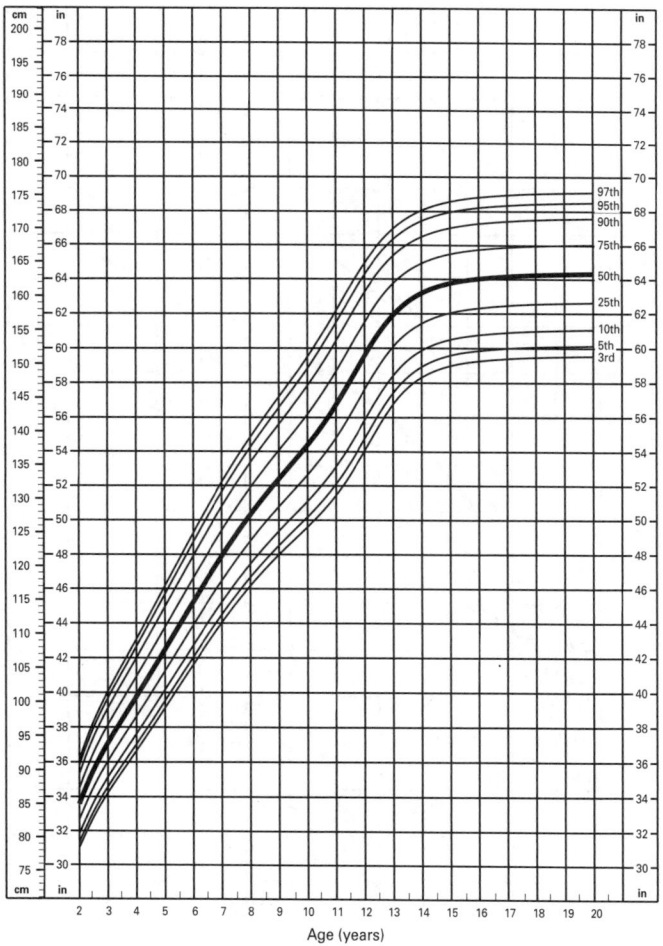

Source: Developed by the National Health Center for Health Statistics in collaboration with the National Center for Chronic Disease Prevention and Health Promotion (2000).

Table 18.5 Weight-for-Age Percentiles, Boys, Birth to 36 Months, CDC Growth Charts: United States

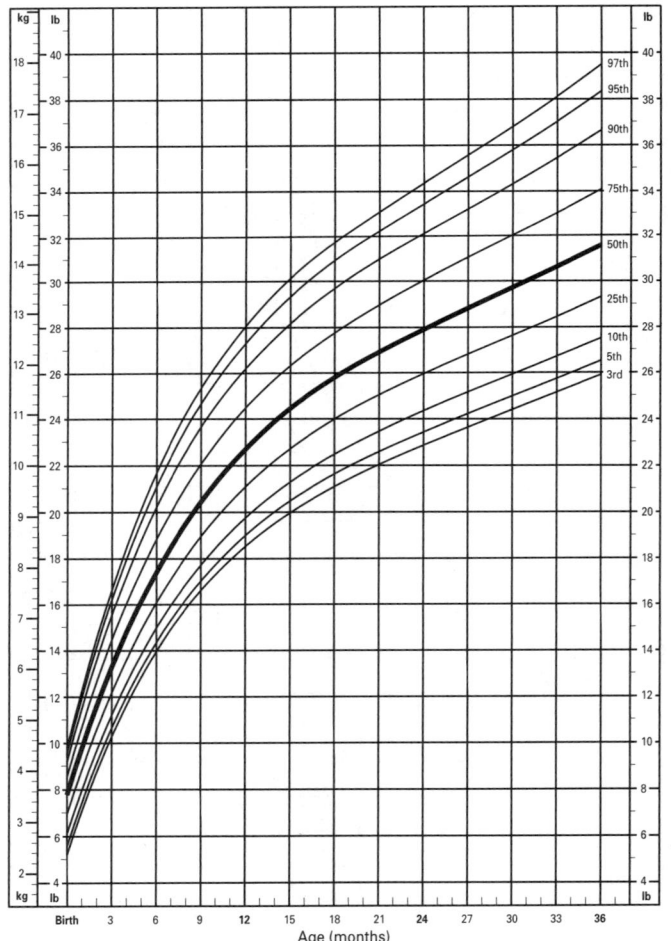

Source: Developed by the National Health Center for Health Statistics in collaboration with the National Center for Chronic Disease Prevention and Health Promotion (2000).

Table 18.6 Weight-for-Age Percentiles, Boys, 2 to 20 Years, CDC Growth Charts: United States

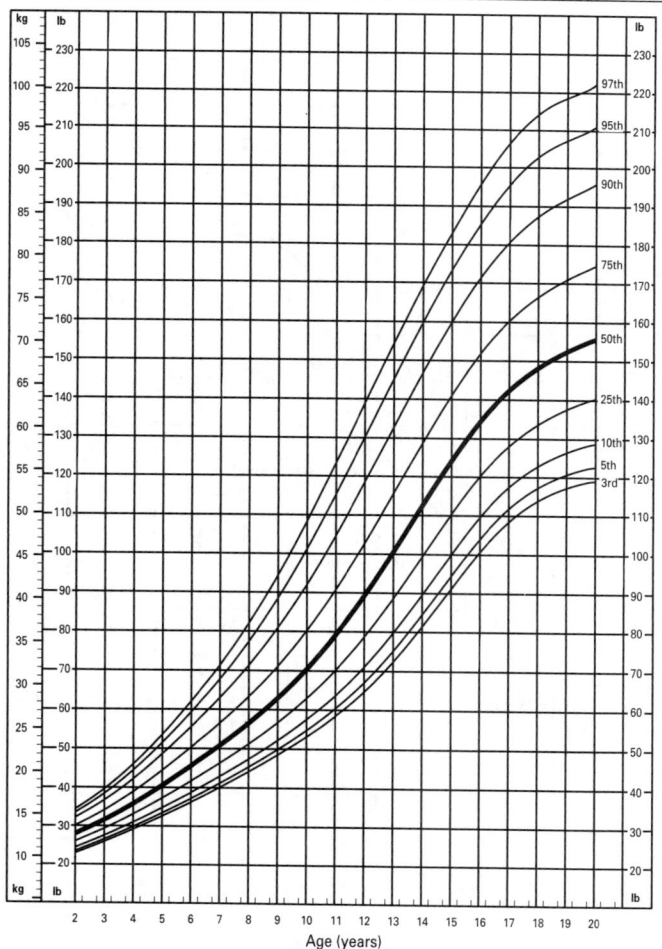

Source: Developed by the National Health Center for Health Statistics in collaboration with the National Center for Chronic Disease Prevention and Health Promotion (2000).

Table 18.7 Weight-for-Age Percentiles, Girls, Birth to 36 Months, CDC Growth Charts: United States

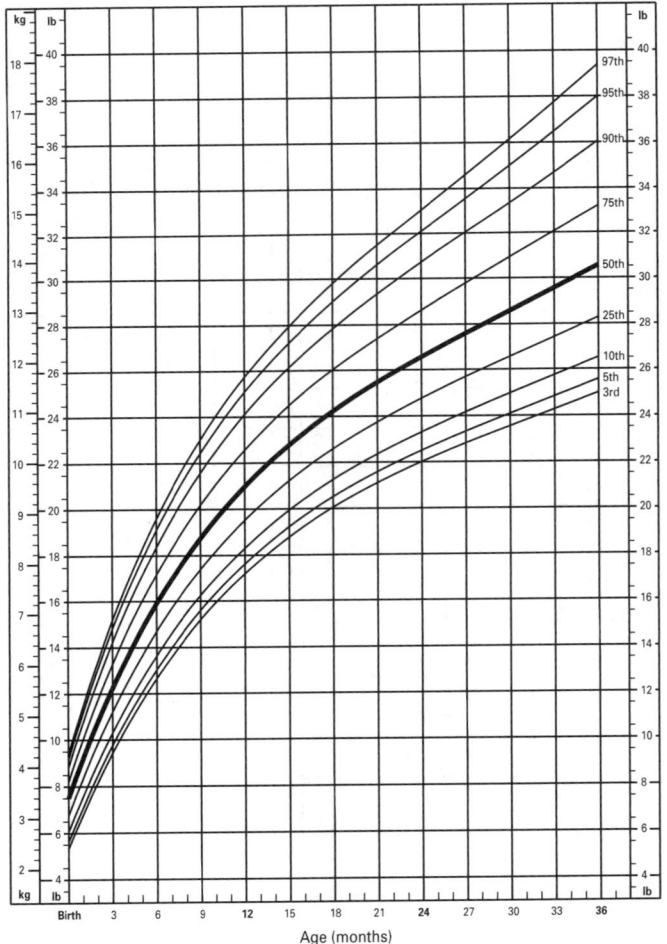

Source: Developed by the National Health Center for Health Statistics in collaboration with the National Center for Chronic Disease Prevention and Health Promotion (2000).

Table 18.8 Weight-for-Age Percentiles, Girls, 2 to 20 Years, CDC Growth Charts: United States

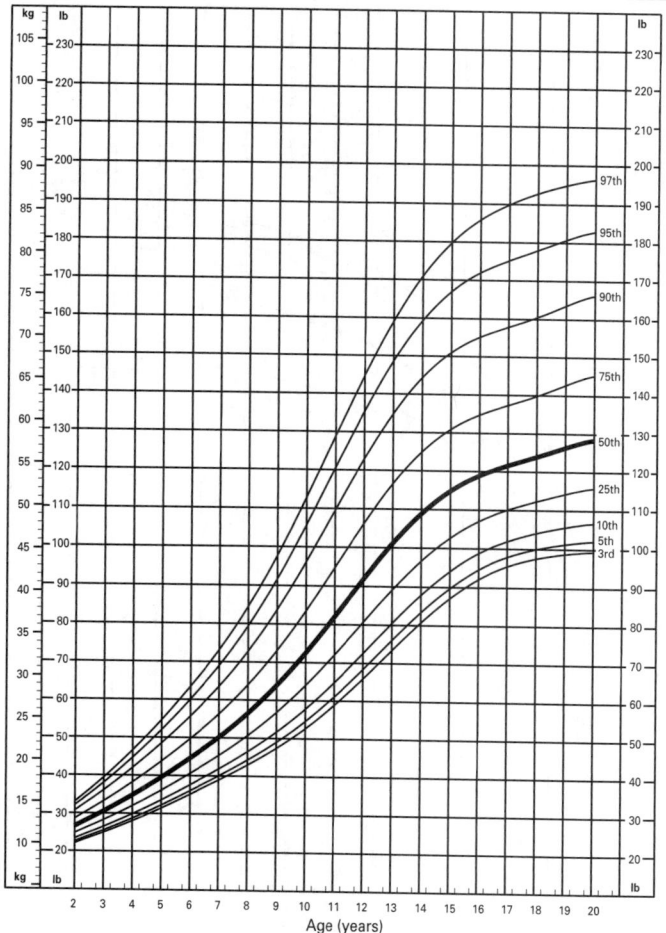

Source: Developed by the National Center for Health Statistics in collaboration with the National Center for Chronic Disease Prevention and Health Promotion (2000).

GROWTH CHARTS

Table 18.9 Head Circumference-for-Age Percentiles: Boys, Birth to 36 Months

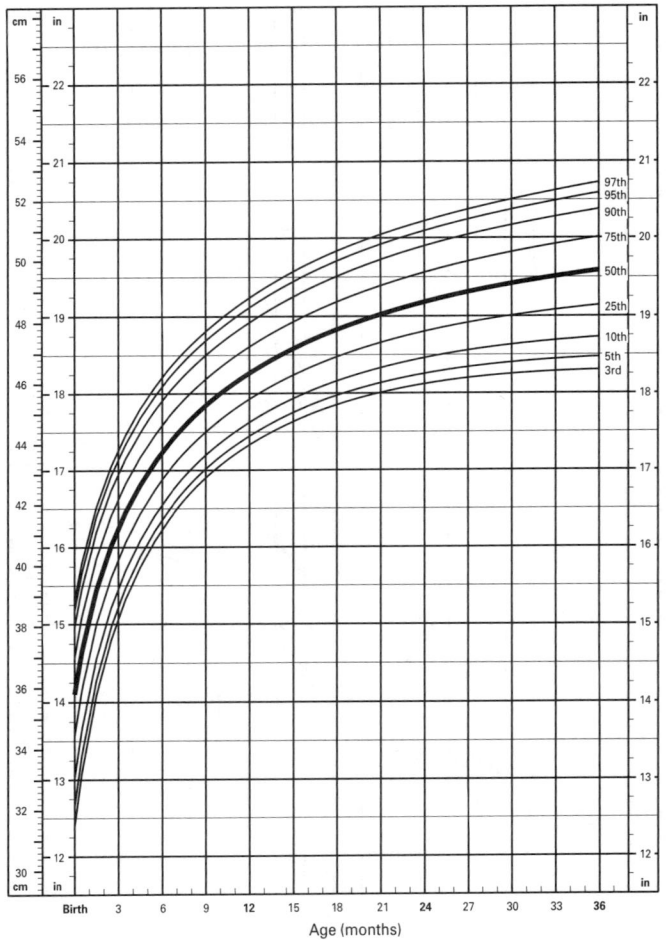

Source: Developed by the National Center for Health Statistics in collaboration with the National Center for Chronic Disease Prevention and Health Promotion (2000).

Table 18.10 Head Circumference-for-Age Percentiles: Girls, Birth to 36 Months

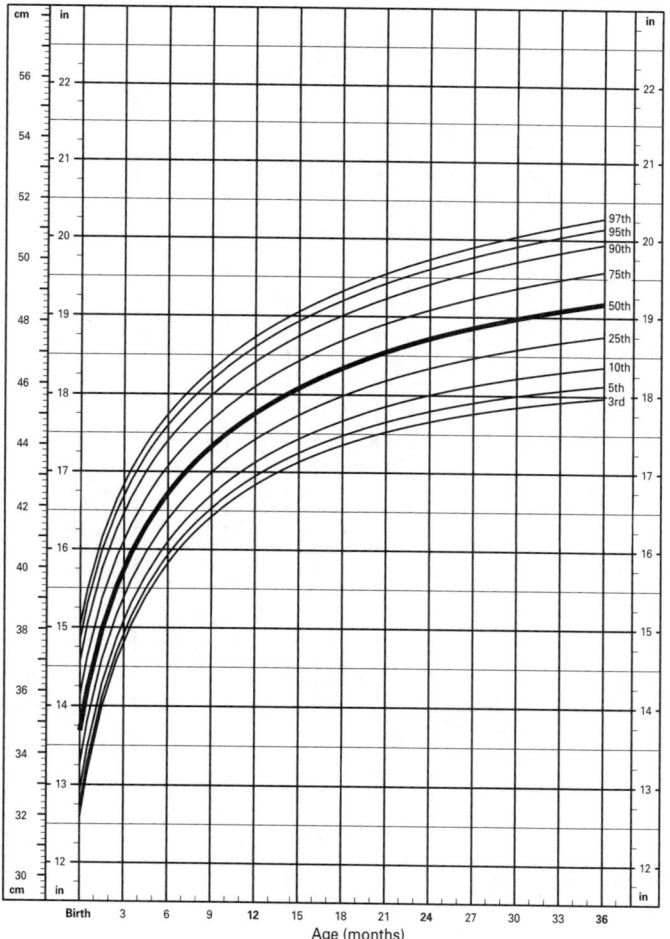

Source: Developed by the National Health Center for Health Statistics in collaboration with the National Center for Chronic Disease Prevention and Health Promotion (2000).

Table 18.11 Body Mass Index-for-Age Percentiles, Boys, 2 to 20 years, CDC Growth Charts: United States

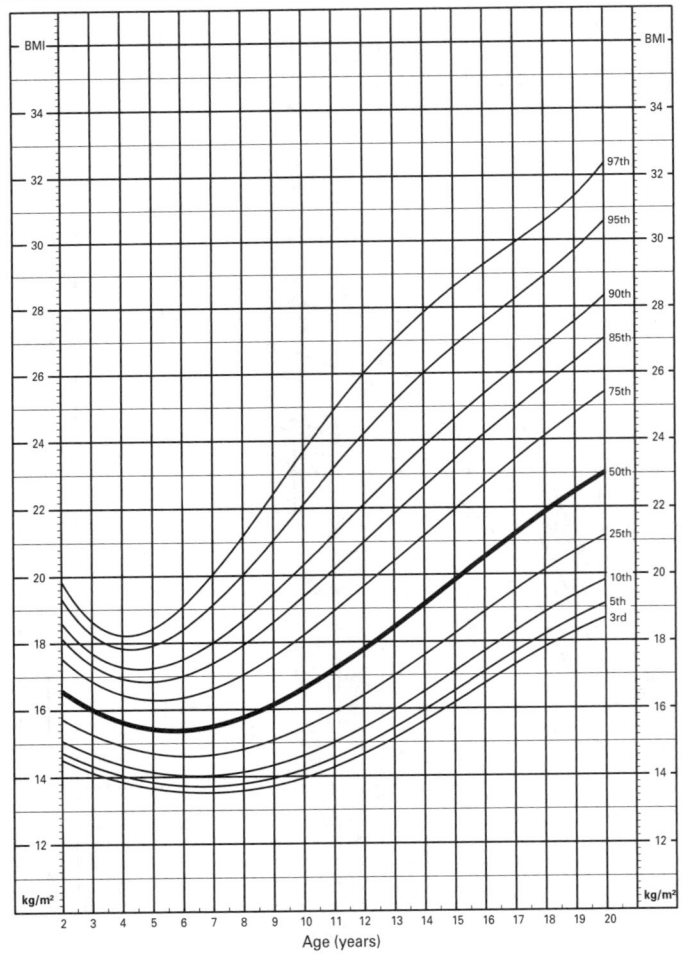

Source: Developed by the National Center for Health Statistics in collaboration with the National Center for Chronic Disease Prevention and Health Promotion (2000).

Table 18.12   Body Mass Index-for-Age Percentiles, Girls, 2 to 20 Years, CDC Growth Charts: United States

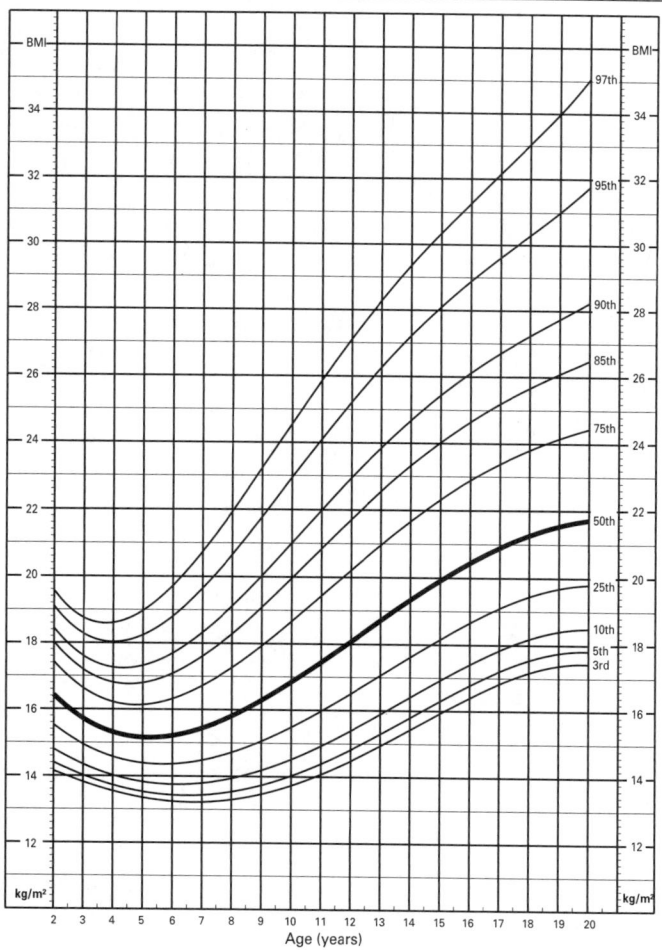

Source: Developed by the National Center for Health Statistics in collaboration with the National Center for Chronic Disease Prevention and Health Promotion (2000).

Index

pyloric stenosis, 101–102

R

RDS (respiratory distress syndrome), 13, 21, 30
recurrent abdominal pain, 126–127
reflux, 124–126
renal tubular acidosis, 137–140
respiratory distress syndrome (RDS), 13, 21, 30
restless legs syndrome (RLS), 207–209, 283
resuscitation, 13–14
retinoblastoma, 320
retinopathy of prematurity, 320
rheumatic fever, 267–268, 309
rheumatology
    acute rheumatic fever, 267–268, 309
    juvenile idiopathic arthritis, 261–264, 309
    systemic lupus erythematosus, 151–152, 264–267, 309
RLS (restless legs syndrome), 207–209, 283
Rocky Mountain spotted fever, 94–95
rolandic epilepsy, 203
rotavirus, 91, 131
RSV (respiratory syncytial virus), 1, 2, 58, 60, 62

S

salmonella, 91
Sarcoptes scabiei, 296
scabies, 296–297
SCFE (slipped capital femoral epiphysis), 310
school refusal, 273
sclerosing cholangitis, 114
seizures, 202–204, 325–327
selective mutism, 273–274
sensorineural hearing loss (SNHL), 33
separation anxiety, 273

sepsis, 14–17
SGA (small for gestational age), 23
shaken baby syndrome, 307
shigella, 91
short stature, 217–219
Shwachman-Diamond syndrome, 164
sickle cell disease, 156, 163–164, 166–169, 309
SIDS (sudden infant death syndrome), 1
sleep apnea, 283
sleep disorders, 281–284
slipped capital femoral epiphysis (SCFE), 310
small for gestational age (SGA), 23
SNHL (sensorineural hearing loss), 33
spina bifida, 340–342
squint, 320–323
Staphylococcus aureus, 79, 80–81
stature-for-age, 357, 359
status asthmaticus, 10–11
stimulants, 271
strabismus, 320–323
strep infections, 95–96
Streptococcus pharyngitis, 76–77
structural lesions, 5
Sturge-Weber syndrome, 205
sudden infant death syndrome (SIDS), 1
suicidal ideation, 275–276
supraventricular tachycardia, 254–255
syncope, 257–258
systemic lupus erythematosus, 151–152, 264–267, 309

T

tall stature, 219–220
TB (total bilirubin), 25
TEC (transient erythroblastopenia), 162
testicular torsion, 38–40
thelarche, 212–213, 215